Teasing Secrets from the Dead

Teasing Secrets

*My Investigations at
America's Most Infamous
Crime Scenes*

from the Dead

Emily Craig, Ph.D.

Foreword by Kathy Reichs

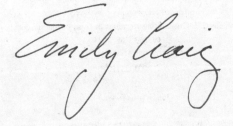

To Debbie — Best Wishes!

Emily Craig

THREE RIVERS PRESS
NEW YORK

Library of Congress Cataloging-in-Publication Data
Craig, Emily A.
Teasing secrets from the dead: my investigations at America's
most infamous crime scenes / by Emily Craig.
1. Forensic sciences. 2. Criminal investigation. 3. Dead—Identification. I. Title.
HV8073.C65 2004
63.25'62—dc22
2003023410

ISBN 1-4000-4923-7

Printed in the United States of America

Design by Leonard W. Henderson

10 9 8 7 6 5 4 3 2 1

First Paperback Edition

To my mother, Emily Josephine,
and to the memory of my father, Reuben.
These two gave me life and the courage to think for myself.

❖　❖　❖

And to the victims,
and the families and friends who loved them.

Contents

FOREWORD BY KATHY REICHS, PH.D. IX

PROLOGUE:
THE STING OF DEATH 1

1

DEATH COMES KNOCKING 14

2

DEATH AND DECAY 43

3

WACO 74

4

CRYING OUT FOR JUSTICE 113

5

A SINGLE DEATH 147

6

FINDING NAMES FOR THE DEAD 184

7

OKLAHOMA CITY 227

8

WORLD TRADE CENTER 241

ACKNOWLEDGMENTS 283

Foreword

by Kathy Reichs, Ph.D.

I CONFESS. It's a puzzler. After working for years in a profession ignored by the masses, my field is suddenly hot.

Don't get me wrong. The disinterest in my science wasn't exclusive to the general public. When I completed graduate school, it was the rare cop or prosecutor who had heard of forensic anthropology. My colleagues and I were a small group back then, known to few, understood by fewer.

Though our numbers have increased over the years, there are still only sixty board-certified practitioners in North America. Along with the military, only a handful of jurisdictions employ full-time anthropologists. The majority of us still serve as external consultants to law enforcement, coroners, and medical examiners.

But our specialty has come of age. Today every TV viewer in America knows who to call for the skeletal, the burned, the decomposed, the mummified, the mutilated, and the dismembered dead.

Ironic. Forensic science is hardly new. The first treatise may have been penned in China in the thirteenth century. In Sung Tz'u's *The Washing Away of Wrongs,* a murder confession is spurred by flies attracted to a bloodstained sickle. Six centuries later, Boston scientist Thomas Dwight documented the use of bones in human identification.

The FBI recognized the value of forensic anthropology early, calling upon Smithsonian scientists for help with human remains. By the first half of the twentieth century, T. Dale Stewart and others were working for the military, examining the bones of American soldiers killed in war.

Forensic anthropology became a formally recognized specialty in 1972, when the American Academy of Forensic Sciences created a Physical Anthropology Section. The American Board of Forensic Anthropology was formed shortly thereafter.

Throughout the seventies, the discipline continued to expand, moving into the investigation of human rights abuses. Spurred by pioneers such as Clyde Snow, anthropologists began digging and setting up labs in Argentina, Guatemala, later Rwanda, Kosovo, and elsewhere. Our role grew in the arena of mass/disaster recovery. Through DMORT (Disaster Mortuary Operational Response Team), we worked plane crashes, cemetery floods, bombings, the World Trade Center.

Still, no one knew our name.

Cue *C.S.I.* The breakthrough sleeper scored millions of TV viewers. Forensic science was suddenly hot, and other series soon followed. *C.S.I.: Miami. Cold Case. Without a Trace.* We'd had *Quincy* in the seventies, but pathology now dazzled. *Crossing Jordan. Da Vinci's Inquest. Autopsy.* Even old-timers such as *Law and Order* and *Dateline* beefed up on ballistics and Y incisions.

True-crime mini-docs weren't far behind. *American Justice. Body of Evidence. City Confidential. Cold Case Files. Exhibit A. Forensic Evidence. Forensic Factor. FBI Files.* All over the airways scientists were slicing and scoping and simulating and solving.

And literature was right in there. Patricia Cornwell. Jeffrey Deaver. Karin Slaughter. And, of course, Kathy Reichs, with my forensic anthropologist heroine, Temperance Brennan.

After decades of anonymity, suddenly we are rock stars.

But the public remains somewhat confused as to the players. What's a pathologist? What's an anthropologist? I am asked the question again and again.

Many fictional scientists are *pathologists*—specialists who work with soft tissue. Emily Craig and I are *anthropologists*—specialists who work with bone. Freshly dead or relatively intact corpse: pathologist. Skeleton in an attic, charred body in a Cessna, bone fragments in a wood chipper: anthropologist. Using skeletal indicators, we address questions of identity, time and manner of death, and postmortem treatment of the corpse.

And we don't work alone. While TV glamorizes the individual heroics of the lone scientist or detective, real-life police work involves cooperation. A pathologist may analyze the organs and brain, an entomologist the insects, an odontologist the teeth and dental records, a molecular biologist the DNA, and a ballistics expert the bullets and casings, while the forensic anthropologist examines the bones. Teamwork is essential. In *Teasing Secrets from the Dead,* Emily accurately portrays the camaraderie and dedication of crime scene technicians, investigative detectives, and lab scientists interacting to solve a case.

I like to think that my own novels have played some small part in raising public awareness of forensic anthropology. I describe my experiences through my fictional character, Temperance Brennan. In *Teasing Secrets from the Dead,* Emily does the same. Through Emily. Chapter by chapter she takes you behind the scenes of real-life cases. As the full-time forensic anthropologist for the Commonwealth of Kentucky she's had many. As a former medical forensic artist, she's had even more.

Emily's background is unique. For fifteen years she worked as a medical illustrator, translating the intricacies of bones and joints into sketches and sculpture. She found her way into forensic anthropology through a request for a facial approximation of an unidentified corpse washed up along the Chattahoochee River. She never looked back.

I've known Emily Craig since she was a Bill Bass graduate student doing research at the University of Tennessee's "Body Farm." In 1998 we coauthored a chapter in my book *Forensic Osteology: Advances in the Identification of Human Remains.* Most recently, Emily and I deployed with DMORT to New York City in the wake of the World Trade Center disaster. While I worked the landfill, Emily worked the ME office. As a veteran of that effort, I appreciate the manner in which her book portrays the dedication of those who took part. The final chapter brought back yet again the horror, the overwhelming sense of mission, and the healing comradeship we all found at Ground Zero.

When I first heard the proposal for *Teasing Secrets from the Dead,* I was skeptical. Could Emily's book acquaint readers with the full spectrum of our discipline and not read like a text? Could she accurately describe methodology, yet bring the human side of our work to life? Could she convey a mother's pain over an absent child, a detective's frustration at an unresolved murder, a sheriff's sorrow at the sight of a bullet-ridden toddler?

The first few chapters put my fears to rest. *Teasing Secrets from the Dead* offers an honest and absorbing snapshot of our profession. Page by page, Emily allows the reader a glimpse over her shoulder and into her thoughts and feelings. Through her stories she provides an understanding of the difficult, demanding, but profoundly rewarding work of a forensic anthropologist.

And, perhaps more poignantly, Emily opens a door to herself as woman and scientist, struggling to balance passion, objectivity, and human vulnerability, to maintain humor and grace in a difficult and often heartrending occupation. *Teasing Secrets from the Dead* captures both the scientific and human sides of forensic anthropology.

Teasing Secrets from the Dead

Prologue
The Sting of Death

I answer the heroic question
"Death, where is thy sting?" with
"It is here in my heart and mind and memories."
— MAYA ANGELOU

I HAD ALREADY spent an inordinate amount of time on the victim's eyes, and I was starting to get frustrated. No matter what I did, I couldn't seem to make her look alive.

Early the day before, I'd propped this woman's head up in the middle of my kitchen table, and I'd been working on it ever since. Now it was two a.m.—long past my usual bedtime—but I just couldn't stop.

Maybe if I worked on another part of the face? I ran my fingers over her cold, smooth cheeks, trying to shake the feeling that her lifeless stare was somehow directed at me. Pressing my thumbs against the soft fold that formed her lower lip, I reshaped her frown into a smile. Then

I realized with a start what I had done. After everything she'd gone through, how in the world could I imagine this woman smiling?

·   ·   ·

My colleagues and I knew far too little about the woman whose face I was attempting to re-create, but what we did know was chilling. About three months before, her remains had been discovered at Peck's Landing, a recreational spot on the Wisconsin River, near the tiny town of Baraboo. A teenager swimming in the river had found a black duffel bag on a sandbar. Thinking it contained camping equipment, he had pulled it over to the trail along the shore. When he opened it, he discovered a plastic trash bag that had come open just enough to disclose the foul-smelling bloody remains of what he assumed was a dead animal. Disgusted, he dumped the plastic-wrapped remains out onto the trail, hung the duffel bag on a nearby tree, and took off. Investigators would have to track him down later to get his story.

That same afternoon, two young brothers were out on their usual Sunday hike along the trail with their mother. They'd gone ahead of her and run into the bloody trash bag. Typical kids, they poked at it with sticks until the plastic tore away and exposed the rotting flesh. They, too, assumed the remains must be from an animal, and they eagerly called their mother over to see what they'd found. She swiftly pulled her kids away and called 911.

When the Sauk County Sheriff's Department determined that the bag contained a human torso, a full-scale search began for additional evidence regarding what was obviously a brutal crime. Over the next few days, searchers found seven more plastic bags full of body parts, each marked with the logo of a local grocery chain. The bags revealed the systematically butchered body parts of a young woman in her twenties—her shoulders, hips, knees, and ankles almost surgically cut apart, her legs literally deboned. She had been decapitated and her skull had been skinned. The face had been completely flayed from the bone.

Ironically, the very steps that the killer had taken to conceal his victim's identity helped preserve it. The plastic bags, neatly tied shut and thrown into the river, had protected their contents much better than had the remains simply been tossed into the woods. Not only had the plastic prevented maggots and other scavengers from eating the flesh, but the river had acted as a refrigerator, slowing the process of natural rot and decay. This young woman's remains still had a story to tell—if only we knew how to hear it.

When Sauk County Homicide Detective Joe Welsch first called me for help, he sounded more discouraged than any detective I'd ever talked to.

"Frankly," Joe began, "this poor girl has been butchered in a way no one up here has ever seen before."

I had the impression that he was young and maybe a little nervous.

"And then there are all those other cases—that woman they found out in New Hampshire, floating in the New Hampshire River, about ten days before ours. Her body was mutilated, too, just like our victim's."

I had also heard about that woman, and I knew that Joe and I were thinking the same thing: serial killer. Such killers are extremely rare, and those of us in the law enforcement community know that they're usually the least likely explanation for any homicide. Still, the sheer brutality of this murder was out of the ordinary. Serial killers like Jeffrey Dahmer and Jack the Ripper seemed unsatisfied to merely kill their victims. The added insult of mutilation or even cannibalism took the act of homicide over the edge of predictable human behavior. This case fit that profile. If Joe had a serial killer in his jurisdiction, he was right to be worried.

"We've already put one serial killer behind bars up here," he went on. "And the folks in Chicago have had twelve women dumped on the streets in the past few months. I've talked to the FBI profiler there, and the one in Madison. We're all trying real hard not to jump to any conclusions. But I'd feel a whole lot better if we could just figure out who this woman is."

Yes, I thought, the clock was ticking. Every minute that we didn't know who this woman was gave the killer one more minute to cover his tracks—or to plan his next murder.

Joe read to me from the autopsy report. "Internal organs and brain, all present—but barely recognizable . . . Teeth all present, and in excellent condition . . . No identifying scars or tattoos . . . No evidence of previously broken bones . . ." This was the standard medical examiner's checklist, and now I understood just how serious Joe's problem was: Virtually nothing about this young woman's body could be used to tell us who she was.

"What about fingerprints?" I asked.

Joe sighed. "Well, we have them, and we don't have them. She had started to decompose by the time we got to her, and after all that time in the water, the skin on her hands was sloughing off."

As a result, Joe told me, his fingerprint expert had had to harden the skin by soaking it in formalin. Then he had teased the epidermis away from the victim's fingertips so that the outer layer of skin could be lifted off in one piece, a maneuver known as de-gloving. The resulting epidermal glove offered a kind of ghostly outline of the victim's fingers, allowing Joe's expert to slip his own fingers, one at a time, into the victim's skin. By rolling each of her fingertips onto an inked pad and a white piece of paper, he had somehow managed to lift six readable prints—a remarkably high number.

"But that's great," I said. It's so difficult to get fingerprints when remains are badly decomposed that I wondered for a moment why Joe sounded so discouraged. Then he reminded me how frustratingly limited fingerprint information can be.

"Yes," Joe said, "but we haven't found any prints that match. You know, when we first got the prints, I thought that all I had to do was enter them into a database. The computer would generate a list of a few missing persons, and bingo! We'd have our woman."

Contrary to popular belief, there is no magic formula for matching the fingerprints of unidentified victims to those of missing persons unless the missing person's fingerprints are already on file in a national or international database. The prints of convicted criminals are usually on file with the arresting agency, but if local police or sheriffs don't submit those prints to a national computerized database, investigators in other jurisdictions can't match them to prints from an unidentified person. Even the most specific biological profiles (age, race, sex, stature, weight, hair color, eye color) can match thousands of missing persons. If investigators haven't included dental records or fingerprints in the missing persons reports they file, then each John or Jane Doe who resembles the victim's biological profile must be examined by hand—and either included or excluded as a possible match.

Usually, you've got a huge stack of printouts, listing all the missing persons on file who might match your victim. The printout gives each person's name, date of birth, date and place of last contact, race, sex, height, weight, hair color, eye color, and hopefully some unique identifiers—clothing worn when last seen; tattoos; scars; birthmarks; missing limbs or digits; old surgeries or fractures; dentures. If finger-prints are available, you might see them in the form of a computerized code. With luck, you'll find a coded version of a dental chart if the original investigating agency has gone to the trouble to get one; if den-tal records or x-rays* are on file somewhere, the printouts may simply say that they're available. The last thing on the list is the name of the submitting agency. It's up to you to contact them if you want to match your unidentified remains with data from their missing person—dental records, fingerprints, DNA, and so forth.

Of course, sometimes the person you're trying to identify never even made it into the database. If she's a loner, perhaps no one missed her enough to call the police. Or maybe the killer is the only one who knows that a certain woman is missing, and *he* certainly won't file a report! I could see why it was so hard for Joe to identify a body with no scars, defects, dental work, or dental records on file.

When I'm in Joe's position, I sit in my lab, looking at the huge stack of printouts, the heart-wrenching descriptions of missing children,

---

*Although technically the product of an x-ray machine is called a radiograph, in this book I'll use the colloquial term "x-ray" to refer to both the process and the product.

spouses, friends, and lovers, and I sometimes have to face the fact that none of them matches the one man or woman whose bones lie there in front of me. Even after all these years, I get that familiar sinking feeling—and then, gradually, a growing sense of determination. Something about being up against an obstacle seems to fill me with a quiet resolve not to be defeated by even the most difficult case.

Still, it can get discouraging sometimes, and lots of investigators simply give up if they don't identify the victim after a few days or weeks. In fact, when I first started working as a forensic anthropologist, I was surprised by how easily some investigators would just move on, letting these cases go unsolved as they quickly grow cold. Over the years, though, I've learned that all you can do is your best during the short time that a case is active—but you never really give up the chase. Now I tease all the secrets I can from "my" unidentified remains, and I make sure that the information is circulated to the public and entered into the system. Then I file it away and hope that someday we'll have an answer as new cases start to demand my attention.

No matter what else I'm working on, though, none of my cold cases are ever really abandoned. Whenever I get any information on a possible match for a John or Jane Doe, I always follow up—I couldn't live with myself if I didn't. Sometimes I think that with an ID system as random as this one, it's a wonder that *any* unknown skeletal remains ever get identified. That's why every single "hit" is such a thrill.

In the end, the Quixote-like nature of our quest may be exactly what keeps me and some of the detectives going. Joe Welsch, for example. Despite his frustration, he was clearly one of these unflagging investigators—he had refused to give up, even in the face of overwhelming odds. He'd joined forces with an equally determined colleague, Special Agent Elizabeth Feagles of the Wisconsin Division of Criminal Investigation—"Liz" to her friends. Together, they'd gone through the usual routine, sorting through the hundreds of missing persons reports, moving from local to state to national cases, but nothing had checked out and they'd run into a wall with the fingerprints, too. They'd gone on to the usual media blitz, bombarding the local news with their best description of Jane Doe—but all they'd gotten for their trouble was a huge stack of false leads.

Three months had passed since the remains had been found, and the killer was still out there. As a last resort, Joe had suggested a facial reconstruction—a clay sculpture representing a forensic artist's rendition of what the victim had looked like. Photographs of the sculpture could then be circulated throughout the state and someone who knew the young woman might recognize her and come forward.

Clay facial reconstructions are always a last-ditch effort—a means of identification employed only when all others have failed. Contrary to popular belief, a facial reconstruction can never be a portrait of the victim, but only, at best, a skillfully rendered approximation. The success of this endeavor is dependent on three things. First, you need a complete and accurate biological profile of the victim. Second, the sculpture must resemble the victim in shape and proportion enough to enable recognition. Third, and most important, someone who knows the victim has to see the reconstruction or a photo made from it. However good the sculpture might be, it does no good at all unless the right person happens to see it.

Joe and Liz were well aware of the difficulties. But what choice did they have? They had to go forward. Then they encountered yet another roadblock.

Usually, a three-dimensional facial reconstruction is built on the skull itself. If some soft tissue still adheres, you actually have to boil the head in a slow cooker—like a Crock-Pot—until the flesh falls away from the bone and you can apply clay directly to the clean, dry contours.

In this case, though, the skull itself couldn't be used. The most critical evidence here was the cut marks, the traces left by the murderer's knife, particularly the marks embedded in the tissue that still clung to the young woman's skull. No one wanted to abandon the possibility that a murder weapon might yet be found to match those marks and the D.A. had insisted that the skull be preserved untouched. But how else could a facial reconstruction be done?

Joe and Liz turned eagerly to the FBI. Surely the forensic specialists at the Bureau, with all their experience, had encountered this problem before? They hadn't. So the investigators contacted Dr. Leslie Eisenberg, a forensic anthropologist and consultant to the medical examiner there in Wisconsin.

Leslie told Joe and Liz about a new technology known as rapid prototyping, a way of creating an exact replica of a human skull without disturbing the head. She also urged them to be cautious. The process was long and complicated, she warned them. It was far from foolproof. And it had never before been employed in the identification phase of a murder case.

Joe and Liz understood that they were breaking new forensic ground. But they'd run out of other options. So they took the now-frozen severed head to their local hospital, where they began the groundbreaking forensic procedure that Leslie had recommended.

First, technicians performed a CT scan on the head, which produced two-dimensional images of the head's structure. Unlike an x-ray, a CT scan can differentiate between skin, muscle, fat, cartilage, bone, and dental components, so it allows the contours of the skull to be clearly delineated.

Then the data identified as "hard tissue" was stored on an ordinary computer diskette, which Joe ferried over to the Milwaukee School of Engineering's Rapid Prototype Center. The engineers there mainly built prototypes of complicated machines and innovative inventions, so this job was something new for them, but they were perfectly capable of using their technology to make an exact scale-model replica of the bones and teeth in Jane Doe's head.

The prototype skull was an amazing piece of work. Made of hundreds of layers of paper that were then laminated with a grayish-brown polyurethane resin, the replica looked exactly like a real skull—until you looked at it up close. Then you could see the layered paper, and the skull resembled a three-dimensional topographical map, a little piece of human geography.

Elated with their success, Joe and Liz went back to the FBI to request a reconstruction using the model skull. But the guys at the Bureau are renowned for their caution, and they just weren't ready to get involved with this new procedure—particularly since neither the FBI's forensic artists nor its consulting anthropologists at the Smithsonian Institution were familiar with the technology used to create the model.

Joe was devastated. But then the FBI agent offered one last suggestion—me.

.   .   .

My name is Emily Craig. I'm the forensic anthropologist for the Commonwealth of Kentucky, a job that usually keeps me plenty busy with our own in-state cases—everything from mysterious bones found in the bed of a mountain creek to a backwoods homicide disguised by fire. My unique background as a medical illustrator and sculptor, along with my years of experience in forensic anthropology, means that special bone cases occasionally come to me from out of state, and, of course, I'm happy to help whenever I can. In fact, it was my earlier career in orthopedics that had made me familiar with the combination of medical and industrial technology used to create the model skull. And it was my forensic anthropology training that had spurred in me a newfound desire to give every victim a name. So when Joe told me the horrifying story of the young woman whose remains he'd found, I was glad that I might have the expertise to help identify her.

I had first learned of this new computer technology a decade earlier when I'd encountered it as an illustrator at the Hughston Orthopaedic Clinic in Columbus, Georgia. We'd sometimes resorted to this very process of bone modeling to help surgeons plan their most demanding surgeries, repairing severe complex fractures. Then, when I first entered graduate school in forensic anthropology at the University of Tennessee, I tapped back into this amazing computer technology and worked up a research proposal for incorporating medical CT-scan technology into the traditional forensic practice of three-dimensional clay reconstruction. I was hoping to come up with a computer pro-gram that could reliably regenerate a person's face from the skull, com-bining the best of art and science. This was one of many times that my background in art and orthopedics and my work in anthropology would turn out to dovetail in unprecedented ways.

I went on to develop the process and to present my preliminary research findings at several international conferences, sparking the interest of the FBI. That's how they'd known to recommend me to Joe: They knew that I'd be on the cutting edge of any technique concern-ing computer-generated faces and CT scans.

But Joe didn't know about any of that background. All he knew was that I was one more scientist who had the power either to take his investigation further or to shut it down once and for all. So he was a little cagey about bringing up the rapid prototyping issue at first. He just started by asking if I might be willing to produce a clay recon-struction of the victim's face.

I wondered why this Wisconsin detective had reached out halfway across the country for a clay reconstruction that he should have been able to get someone to do right in his own home state. Then Joe explained that this job involved not only creating a standard forensic facial sculpture but also working with a computer-generated prototype skull—a job that even the FBI's experts weren't quite confident enough to take on. When I told him I'd do the job anyway, he was elated. As soon as I said I could do the work over the upcoming holiday week-end, he promised to get into his car the very next day so he could hand-deliver the skull replica to me that Friday evening.

Usually, facial reconstruction projects require close collaboration between a forensic sculptor and a forensic anthropologist, but I'm one of the few people who happen to be both. So there I was, alone in my kitchen at two a.m., trying to make a young woman's face come alive with nothing to go on but a laminated paper skull and a set of mathe-matical formulas telling me the average tissue depths for the face of a young Black woman. I'd played it safe to that point, using tiny erasers to mark the tissue depths and then covering them with clay, arranging the eyes and nose according to standard scientific guidelines. But those hard, cold data weren't enough. My reconstruction didn't yet resemble an actual human being enough to prompt anyone to recognize her. I knew I would have to let my intuition take over in order to bring this sculpture alive.

Slowly my hands took on a life of their own. Following some secret instructions, an intuitive sense of the subtleties of facial structure, my fingertips began exploring the contours of the victim's face. I shut my eyes, relying entirely on my sense of touch.

For a moment, I thought I had something. Then my hands dropped to my sides and I opened my eyes. A headache started to press against my temples as I sat there, frustrated, my statue staring blankly back at me.

Then, without having consciously planned to do so, I found myself reaching out to her left eyelid, tweaking its clay surface ever so slightly. Just that tiny adjustment made her finally begin to look alive. Suddenly, I knew exactly what to do next. Saturating a cotton ball with isopropyl alcohol, I rubbed it across the glass eyes I had inserted, trying to remove the greasy residue left by the clay. As the irises cleared and the corneas brightened, those eyes began to reflect the room light, as real human eyes do. Better. Much better.

Moving more quickly then, I dripped more alcohol into the inside corner of each eye, until large pools formed in the depression where the woman's tear ducts would have been. Slowly, the drops welled up and spilled over, running down the edges of her nose and into the corners of her mouth. She appeared to be crying—which was just what I wanted.

This macabre effect is one of my secret recipes, a way to test the accuracy of the topography of the mid-face area, between the eyebrows and the mouth. When tears fall from a real person's eyes, they follow a fairly predictable pattern down both sides of the face. If a reconstruction is even slightly off, its "tears" will flow erratically, curving back and forth in an odd snakelike effect, or following two irregular routes down each side of the nose. These tears flowed just as human ones do, and watching them flow down her cheeks, I felt my own tears slowly well up. As a scientist, I try hard to stay emotionally detached while I'm working on a case. I make an effort to "think like a murderer" rather than to identify with the victims. But that night I was exhausted, and when that last procedure made the face of that sculpture spring to life, I surprised myself. This woman had been butchered like an animal, and I hadn't yet even allowed myself to truly think of her as a person. She suddenly had a face—a young, innocent face—and the horror of what she had been through overcame me.

•   •   •

As the forensic anthropologist for the Commonwealth of Kentucky, my job is to analyze bones, fragments of extremities, and charred human remains, helping to determine how people died, who they were, and sometimes even what they looked like. On any given day, you might find me beside the smoking wreckage of a plane crash, sifting the ashes of a burned-down backwoods cabin, or in my lab, carefully cataloguing a suspicious-looking pile of bones. I'm often the one to tell the pathologist whether we're looking at homicide or accident, and the evidence I collect might prove crucial in helping investigators decide upon their next step. Sometimes, I'm the detectives' last chance to find a killer or the family's final hope for closure in the loss of a missing loved one.

It can be gruesome, but I love my job. I thrive on the challenge of solving a mystery, of working with complex puzzles that call upon every ounce of my wit and resourcefulness. I cherish the men and women with whom I work, and I feel honored to be accepted as one small part of the team of law enforcement and medical workers who strive so hard to bring justice into the world. That mission, above all, is what drives me, even when I'm working late into the night on a seemingly hopeless case.

It's taken me half my life to find this work that I love so much. My first profession was as a medical illustrator, working with Dr. Jack

Hughston as he developed pioneering surgical techniques in sports medicine. I was proud of the contributions I had made to the work of surgeons and researchers, but after two decades of creating sketches, models, and computer-generated animation, I started looking for a way to become a scientist in my own right. When a detective I happened to be dating started telling me about his cases, I became intrigued with the world of law enforcement. When his recommendation led to my creating a facial reconstruction of an unidentified homicide victim, I was hooked.

Coping with the aftermath of violent human behavior has its rewards, but also its pitfalls. From the moment I entered the world of murder investigations, I had to learn that my life was no longer my own. I would be on call twenty-four hours a day, seven days a week, through holiday weekends and times that had theoretically been set aside for vacation.

There were emotional demands as well. If I was truly to understand what had happened to the men and women whose remains I handled, I had to understand the depravity of human violence that had led to their deaths. I was sucked down into this vortex of murderous hate and malice each time I dealt with mutilated body parts and skeletal remains of murdered victims.

Still, it's been an exhilarating journey, and I wouldn't change it for the world. I've crawled deep into Kentucky coal mines and clung to the rock faces of steep mountains. I've worked lonely murders out in the backwoods and mass disasters in the centers of major cities. I've met killers who turned themselves in to the authorities so they could get free medical care from prison doctors, and I've brought comfort to survivors who refused for decades to give up hope of finding out what happened to their missing loved ones. My cases have ranged from the tragic to the downright bizarre, from the awe-inspiring to the purely depressing, but my profession is now my passion: the ultimate challenge—and the ultimate reward.

1

Death Comes Knocking

Pale Death with impartial tread beats at the
poor man's cottage door and at the palaces of kings.

— H O R A C E

M Y FIRST CASE STARTED just as so many cases begin for me
today—with an unidentified victim. A couple of bass fish-
ermen had found some decomposed and partially skeletonized remains on the edge of West Point Lake, one of the huge
Chattahoochee River impounds that separate the lower portions
of Alabama and Georgia. The man had been shot in the head and his
body had washed up onto the riverbank. The Georgia Bureau of
Investigation (GBI) had been working the case, but after several weeks,
they still had no identification for the victim, and it looked as if this
murder might be headed for the cold-case files.

I was still a civilian then, a medical illustrator at a nearby orthopedic clinic, but the police thought I might be able to help by doing a clay facial reconstruction of the victim. When police officers escorted me into the forensic morgue for the first time, I had my first whiff of the smell of decayed human flesh. It was like nothing I'd ever experienced, and I felt an overpowering sense of repulsion. Yet I was also drawn to the mass of bone and decaying tissue that once had been a man—I'd never seen anything like it before. It was slimy and grayish, with bits of bone and rotting leaves and twigs sticking up randomly from a form that I could still recognize as human—but this form had flattened, melted into the black vinyl of the body bag.

As the investigators began to tell me what they knew, I was amazed at how much they'd already learned simply from examining the remains. Enough pelvic soft tissue remained to reveal that this victim was a man; and the coroner, Don Kilgore, had estimated his height from the size label sewn into the trouser remnants that still clung to his leg bones. Now Don gently held the head, which had decomposed down to bare bone, and he showed me the bullet hole, explaining how he could tell where the bullet had entered the man's head, and at what angle. Don had been lucky: He'd recovered a .45-caliber bullet from inside the skull. If police could only link a suspect to the victim, they might be able to solve the crime by comparing bullet evidence.

But the first step, as in every murder investigation, was to identify the victim. Don pointed to some fillings in the man's teeth. If they could just get someone to suggest a name for the victim, he told me, they could probably match the man's teeth to a missing person's dental records. They were starting to lose hope, though. This victim's remains had been here in the morgue for way too long already, and so far no one had come forward with a name.

That's where I came in. At the time, I was dating a detective, Brian McGarr, and all I knew of crime was what I'd heard from him, as he kept me up nights with long, grisly stories of his latest homicide cases. He, in turn, had the incredible good luck to hear all about my exciting work as a medical artist and sculptor, which he at least had the good grace to pretend to find fascinating. Still, maybe he was more interested than I thought. When the West Point case continued to go unsolved, he was the one to suggest to the GBI and the Muscogee County coroner that they commission me to do the facial reconstruction that might help them identify their victim.

Brian and I had a relationship that nicely blended the personal and the professional. He was able to share with me confidential information about police work because I was a volunteer emergency medical technician (EMT) on the local ambulance squad, which gave me an insider's knowledge of the grisly facts surrounding some of his murder cases. Both Brian and I had spent time in the privileged zone behind the yellow crime scene tape, so we understood that unauthorized release of confidential information was forbidden. Still, when professional ethics allowed, we would sit on my back porch for hours hammering out different scenarios that could have caused specific injuries. Sometimes we'd even act out the cases, taking turns playing "killer" and "victim." When Brian had to testify in court, I'd help him mentally prepare by acting as devil's advocate, pummeling him with questions that challenged his findings at the crime scene. I could also add anatomical facts that supported—or, sometimes, refuted—his interpretation of the victim's fatal injuries. Those conversations were where I first learned to think like a detective. I like to think that, at the same time, Brian was learning to think like a scientist.

Certainly, when it came to analyzing a crime scene and events that led to a murder, Brian was the undisputed expert. But once he realized that my formal training as a medical illustrator enabled me to figure out bullet trajectories and other injury patterns just by reading the autopsy reports, he knew my input was just as valuable as his. At the time, I had no idea that these late-night conversations were actually expanding my understanding of human anatomy and laying the groundwork for a future in forensic anthropology and law enforcement.

A few months before, I'd had my first experience as part of a law enforcement team. Brian had recommended me to do a drawing for an upcoming murder trial. This drawing became a pivotal piece of evidence, enabling prosecutors to demonstrate the pattern of a victim's stab wounds: The injured man was defending himself, not initiating an attack, as the murderer claimed. The D.A. won his case.

It was a heady experience for me, as well. To produce my drawing, I'd been given access to confidential information, and I even became involved with prosecution strategy. The excitement was intoxicating, and I found myself rethinking my current career as a medical illustrator, which began to seem humdrum and predictable by comparison. Brian knew how much I'd come to yearn for something new and exciting, which may have been why he recommended me for the facial reconstruction job.

Still, flattered though I was, I wanted to say no. An anatomical drawing for a trial was one thing. But a sculpture for an ongoing investigation? First of all, I wasn't trained in the technique. Second, this was serious stuff. If I got it wrong, I might ruin their last chance to crack the case.

I wanted to help, though, and I thought I could at least do a little liaison work. So I called Betty Pat Gatliff, a friend and medical illustrator who was also one of the world's best-known forensic sculptors. Her lectures at conferences had fascinated me for years. I'd hung on her every word as she described her work in helping to identify some of the twenty-eight victims of the serial killer John Wayne Gacy, as well as victims of the Green River Killer. One of her first success stories concerned a young Native American who had disappeared years before. Betty Pat produced a facial reconstruction that bore an incredible likeness to the victim and led to the man's positive identification. This brought her more referrals from medical examiners across the country.

On one referral, she actually used her knowledge of human skulls to uncover a flaw in the initial investigation. Skeletal remains and the victim's clothing had been discovered in a remote section of the Southwest, and the victim's bra, lace panties, and high-heeled pumps were collected along with the bones. Naturally, the detectives assumed the victim was female. But when Betty Pat was brought in to do one of her now-famous facial reconstructions, she realized that the skull may have actually belonged to a man. Further forensic anthropology analysis proved her right, and the detectives went on to identify the remains as those of a man who secretly cross-dressed and who had apparently been killed when a prospective lover discovered the deception.

Now, when I approached Betty Pat about the West Point case, she was just as pleasant as I'd remembered—but not very encouraging. "My plate is fuller than full," she said apologetically. "I couldn't get to this case for at least a year. Why don't you take my course and do it yourself?"

Me? Attend a workshop on forensic sculpture? I was working full-time at a clinic specializing in sports medicine. How could I fit a whole other course of study into my schedule? Still, I was intrigued—and tempted. I haltingly told Betty Pat that I'd think about coming to her class, not realizing how much that conversation would change my life.

.   .   .

Looking back, I realize that, in many ways, my talk with Betty Pat was merely the next step in a journey I'd been on since childhood. For as long as I can remember, I have been blessed—or maybe cursed—with an insatiable curiosity about the human body. Call me crazy, but my idea of a good time is a pile of mysterious bones to analyze, the chance to dissect the bloody knee of a freshly delivered cadaver, or maybe a long session of photographing a partially decayed face—anything to satisfy my endless fascination with the form and function of our bones, muscles, and tendons.

As a girl growing up in Kokomo, Indiana, in the 1950s and 1960s, I was discouraged from choosing a career in science, as well as from engaging in other kinds of "boy stuff." So my fascination with science made me feel like a misfit, though given my family history, it should have made sense: My dad, *his* dad, and my mother's grandfather had all been doctors. How could I help myself?

My father's medical books especially fascinated me. I got his permission to take them off his library shelves—and became hooked. Looking through those books, I felt as though I had entered into another world. I spent hours admiring the full-color renderings of what I might see inside an arm, a leg, or an abdomen. Although he never expected me to make a career in science or medicine, Dad encouraged my interest in those books. I guess he was thrilled that he could share his passion for anatomy with at least one of his four kids.

One afternoon when I was about twelve, I was out in a trout stream near a vacation cabin we owned near Baldwin, Michigan. Suddenly, I caught sight of some bones sticking out of the sandy bank. At that point in my life, it took quite a lot for me to put down my fly rod voluntarily, especially when the trout were biting. But those bones were just too intriguing. I waded over to the bank and pulled a few out of the sand. Just below, under the water, I could see that more were deeply embedded in the black muck just below the surface of the streambed. I was sure that I had stumbled upon a deer's antlers, some ribs, and a pelvis. That was it. I knew I couldn't leave until I had found every single piece of that skeleton.

As I searched for the smooth butter-colored bones among the rocks and sticks at the bottom of the creek, I completely lost track of time. When I suddenly realized that it was starting to get dark, I knew my parents would be frantic. I stuffed all the bones that would fit into my wicker creel, the basket for carrying the fish I'd caught, and thrust the others into a sack I had improvised out of my rain poncho. I reached the path back to our cabin in record time, just as my dad showed up to look for me.

Before Dad could scold me for being late, I dumped the bones at his feet and breathlessly asked him to help me reassemble them, figuring that any doctor could put a skeleton together without thinking twice. But Dad had no idea where to start. He knew where every bone was located while *in* the body, but assembling skeletons hadn't been part of his training. Out of context, the bones just didn't make any sense to him.

That was one time my dad couldn't help me. But he was wise enough to see that I had found something that was hugely important to me. Even though it was nearly twilight, Dad walked me back to my fishing spot and waited quietly on the bank while I finished doing my first-ever skeletal excavation. Then he offered moral support for the next two days, as I tried to put those bones back together in our back-yard.

Of course, I couldn't do it. But I promised myself that someday, somehow, I *would* put a skeleton back together—and a human skeleton, too, not just an animal one.

·   ·   ·

Deer bones from a trout stream were one thing, but I'll never forget the shock of my first encounter with a human cadaver. It was a dozen years later, and I'd enrolled in the medical illustration program at the Medical College of Georgia, where studying the innards of the human body was part of the program. As I walked into the brightly lit gross anatomy lab, I had to blink a bit to avoid the relentless glare of the overhead fluorescent lights. Everything was cold, clean, and sparkling—gleaming stainless steel fixtures, glass cabinets full of lab instruments, and a shiny-white tile floor. I shivered inside my new white lab coat, partly from the cold—the lab was kept air-conditioned to a chilly 68 degrees—and partly from excitement. There were about thirty-five of us, a mix of med students and illustrators, divided ran-domly into groups of five or six, and we were all nervous.

I was naïvely expecting to see the bodies laid out on gurneys in quiet repose, anticipating a funeral home kind of quiet in the lab. Instead, everyone was chattering as the sharp smell of formaldehyde assaulted us. A half-dozen stainless steel coffin-like boxes were scattered around the room, mounted on legs that brought them up to tabletop height.

I went to join my group, and as class began, the four lab instructors went from box to box, flipping back the lids to reveal the cadavers floating there in formalin. The intense smell scoured the lining of my nostrils, bringing tears to my eyes. I blinked and peered into our vat. There was our cadaver—a White woman who looked to be about sixty or seventy years old. She was nude, of course, but for some reason that surprised me. She lay face-up on the bottom of the vat, completely submerged in the cloudy fluid, her flaccid, wrinkled skin hanging in thick folds from her short, square frame. Her sagging flesh was light gray, and her long, wispy silver hair was floating just under the liquid's surface, drifting over her face. Her colorless lips were drawn back from her teeth in a deathly grimace and her eyes were open slightly, exposing ghostly white globes. Apparently her eyes had sunk back into the sockets after death, and her slightly closed lids hid the irises. It was a ghoulish sight, but my insatiable scientific curiosity overcame my initial squeamishness.

Around me, the room slowly filled with an uncomfortable silence as one by one the students stopped talking. We had all prepared for this day with such excitement—so proud of our new lab coats, our very own surgical gloves, the little dissection kits we had bought according to our printed instruction sheets—but now we realized how unprepared we really were.

As the conversation quieted, I could hear the low rumble of the exhaust fans sucking the heavy formalin fumes out of the air. Across the room, someone bumped into a stainless steel container and a half-opened lid crashed down. The sound bounced off the tile floor and echoed through the room like a gunshot. Everyone jumped and then laughed self-consciously.

Having opened the containers, the instructors then pulled back on huge stainless steel levers at each end of the vats to lift the bodies up out of the fluid, raising them to table height. I watched transfixed as my group's cadaver rose up slowly, horror movie style, to break through the surface of the oily liquid. Her hair fell back like a swimmer's would while rising out of a pool and then there she lay, stretched out on a perforated steel sheet, the formalin dripping off her body down into the vat. I had the feeling that her most intimate secrets were being revealed: the muted old surgical scar that marked her abdomen; the coarse, dark stubble running up and down her legs; her long, split, and dirty nails. When our instructors told us to flip our cadavers onto their stomachs, I was relieved that I wouldn't have to look into her face any longer, at least not for a while.

It took me a while to overcome the sense that I was trespassing, staring at this woman's most intimate bodily secrets. I was grateful when the instructor started giving instructions on how we were to begin our dissections. Now I didn't have to feel like some sleazy voyeur—I had a purpose for examining this woman's body.

My strongest reaction was that the cadavers were shockingly gray and stiff, so far from the lifelike multicolored tissue I'd expected to explore. During my childhood of hunting and fishing with Dad and my brothers, I had cleaned and dressed plenty of fish and game, and I'd been expecting our specimens in human dissection to be more like that freshly killed tissue—soft, pliable, brightly colored. Working on this washed-out corpse felt like abandoning color TV to watch in black and white. The cadavers' grayness did help with the queasiness of working on a human, though.

We started the dissection by removing the skin, which felt like cold, stiff, waterlogged shoe leather. It had simply not occurred to me that I would have to *skin* a human being. At least the gray, rubbery covering of our cadaver didn't look or feel anything like real human skin. Of course, I was wearing rubber gloves, which added to the eerie sensation. I didn't know it at the time, but I would never touch dead human soft tissue without the feel of latex stretched taut across my fingertips.

Despite the medical touch added by the gloves, I felt as though I were violating this woman. To combat this sensation, my fellow students and I did what we could to depersonalize our cadavers. We didn't give them names, and we referred to each one as "the body" rather than as the "dead person." When I became a forensic anthropologist, I would have to learn how to reverse this line of thought, remembering that each dead body was actually a person with a story to tell. But I wasn't so philosophical back then. Instead, I was consumed by my fascination with the human body. My only response to this dead woman was excitement at the prospect of all she was about to teach me.

My fellow students and I were totally silent as we took turns making the incisions on the woman's back that would allow us to open the skin as if opening a book: first a long cut down the backbone, then a right-angle cut across her shoulders, then another right-angle cut at the base of her spine, just above the crack in her buttocks, to make a giant letter "I." The skin on her back was several layers thick, attached to the tissue underneath with hundreds of little fibers that we had to cut through.

Having spent so much time with my dad's textbooks, I expected to be able to look at a real body and see all the parts clearly, but I soon discovered this wasn't possible. Indeed, that's why medical illustrators are necessary. A medical illustration needs to show fully detailed anatomical structures, something that a surgeon might use to navigate an actual body. But neither the illustrator nor the surgeon ever really sees those complete structures, not all at once. We had to be able to see each layer of the body as we dissected it, then imagine what it all looked like when it was intact and in place.

That's why our instructors insisted that we cut into the body with the "I" shape they had chosen. They wanted us to be able to open the body, remove the organs, and then fold everything back exactly the way it was. If we just cut things out and discarded them as we went along, we'd never see the whole picture. Instead, we had to learn both the parts *and* the whole, both the individual structures and the way they fit together, so that we could someday make illustrations that would enable doctors and surgeons to have their own limited view of the body while visualizing the whole.

The medical students were going through a similar process. It was the only chance they'd get to see a body in layers, or to cut out an organ, trace its blood supply, and then put the dissected pieces back together like some three-dimensional jigsaw puzzle. During actual surgery, their goal would be to disturb as little of the body as possible, imagining—with the help of our illustrations—what they could not actually see.

After we had finished exploring the muscles, nerves, and blood vessels in our cadavers' backs, our instructors finally let us turn them face up. (My group immediately put a paper towel over our woman's face, covering her staring eyes and grinning mouth.) As we cut into the abdomen, I again expected to see what I'd seen in my dad's textbooks: the abdominal organs revealed as separate structures, each with its own unique size and shape. Instead, what I saw was that every organ was molded and folded tightly onto its neighbors, like one of those amazing Irish stone fences, in which a collection of separate stones somehow fit so closely together that mortar isn't necessary.

Sorting through loops of intestines, I realized that they are not just one long tube, like a garden hose, folded over to fit neatly into someone's belly. Instead, they are connected to the body's main blood vessels by huge, flat membranes, which, if torn or twisted, can rob the gut of blood and lead to someone's death. Then I was struck by how huge her liver was—about the size and weight of a wet, tightly folded bath towel. I knew that if I slipped my fingers around the liver's narrow edge, I'd find the gall bladder, tucked up underneath one of the liver's lobes. Since gall bladder removal is a pretty common surgical procedure, we students eventually made it a game to see whether we could tell by feel which cadavers had had that type of surgery.

The nervous system was particularly difficult for me to learn. Among other things, nerve pathways cross and crisscross at specific places in the brain and spinal cord. When the pathways are disrupted—from disease, stabbing, gunshot wounds—the whole system can be short-circuited. It took a leap of faith for me to understand that a gunshot wound that completely pulverized one section of the brain might leave the victim alive but severely disabled, while another gunshot wound that cut cleanly through the brain stem meant instant death as the diaphragm and heart quit forever.

Although at the time I was merely learning the architecture of the human interior in order to draw it accurately, one day this training would be vital for my work in forensics. Years later, while testifying in a murder trial, I became recognized as a court-qualified expert in gross anatomy as well as forensic anthropology—a rare distinction for a forensic anthropologist, and one I could not have achieved without my early studies at the Medical College. The case in question hinged on a minuscule cut in the victim's neck bone no bigger than an eyelash. I was able to prove that the tiny trace mark indicated a fatal knife wound when I demonstrated that in order to reach the bone in question, the killer's knife had to work its way through the victim's windpipe, esophagus, and a critical group of arteries, nerves, and veins.

Those nerves and blood vessels sure caused me enough trouble as a student! When I'd first looked at Dad's textbooks, I'd seen that each body part was rendered in a different color—red for arteries, yellow for nerves, and blue for veins. In real life, though, the colors seemed blurred and dulled, and all I could see were bunches of vessels, tangled together like three incredibly long varieties of overcooked pasta.

Gradually, I got used to the lack of color, and I learned to work by touch as well as by sight. When I could see the organs for myself and follow their contours with my hands, I could memorize their anatomy through my fingertips as the shape and location of even the tiniest lymph node flowed effortlessly from my hands into my brain.

In the anatomy lab, I had the luxury of being able to take bodies apart, piece by piece, to see exactly what made things work. Making my cadaver's fingers wiggle and her knees bend by pulling on a tendon imitated a muscle contraction. It might make this dead woman look like a macabre life-size marionette, but it taught me more than any textbook ever could.

The wonder of those first few months stays with me to this day. I walked around in a perpetual state of awe, amazed at the infinite variety of us humans and our bodies, even as I marveled at how alike we all are. I found myself looking at the crowds of people in the local shopping mall, people of different ages, races, and sizes, thrilled at my new knowledge that each anatomical structure shared a common shape, location, and function. Touch the inside of a wrist—anybody's wrist—and you'll feel the pulse of the radial artery in the same tiny spot . . . every time . . . in every body. This "human design element" is what makes modern forensic science possible—the fact that we know so much about any individual body before we've ever seen it.

Gross anatomy class was also where I learned that you must never—
never—discuss "the bodies" in front of outsiders. You never knew who
might be acquainted with the person whose body you were discussing,
or who might accidentally overhear the conversation. What if your
casual joking was heard by someone whose father had donated his body
to science? How might the listener feel hearing you and your fellow
med students blowing off steam by making derisive remarks about one
of your cadavers? I'm grateful for the lesson now, since the same rule
applies to forensic investigations: You talk about them only with fellow
investigators. I think that's one reason why cops and forensic specialists
maintain such a closed society. Only among our own can a case be discussed openly and freely, without fear of inadvertently wounding a
grieving friend or family member.

This was also when I first encountered the peculiar balancing act that
is the hallmark of my profession: Dead bodies are treated as objects to
be probed for clues—and yet they must also be viewed as the living
human beings they once had been, humans whom we try to honor by
learning who they were and how they died. When I first started working in forensic anthropology, I'd approach each case like a puzzle, and
I spoke only of "the body" or "the bones." When I finally learned to
refer instead to "the dead person" or "the human remains," I was better able to hold on to my sense of each victim's humanity. Out in the
field, it's easy to get wrapped up in the act of searching for bones, teeth,
and evidence associated with the victim—jewelry, clothing, maybe a
bullet—and it's all too common to find yourself shouting gleefully
when someone finds one of these "treasures." Among cops and other
forensic specialists, it probably doesn't matter too much, but the effect
can be devastating when civilians are looking on. I've learned to make
a habit of acting as if the victim's mother were always looking over my
shoulder and treating every piece of tissue, every scrap of evidence, as
if I had a personal connection to the victim.

This approach really paid off when I was working with the remains
of the people who died in the World Trade Center. Then, my every

move really was under scrutiny by dozens of people, often including the victims' friends, families, and fellow firefighters or police officers. I was thankful, then, that I'd learned to treat every human remain with the respect it deserved, and I was moved by how much my colleagues in the morgue appreciated my gentleness and care.

·　　·　　·

As I continued with my medical illustration class, I was most fascinated observing surgical procedures. The medical illustration program at the Medical College of Georgia is considered one of the best in the nation, and one thing that makes it so special are classes in surgical observation, where students get to sketch actual operations while standing at the surgeon's elbow.

Writing these words today, I'm struck by how different my first surgical experience was from those of students today, who have access to television and movies that depict surgery in relatively realistic ways. The closest I'd ever gotten to an operating room before I observed my first surgery was TV's *Ben Casey* and *Marcus Welby, M.D.* In true 1970s television style, I imagined surgery as taking place in cathedral silence, amidst an atmosphere of high seriousness, with reverent doctors and obedient nurses clad in spotless white coats and immaculately clean rubber gloves. I simply had no idea of how bloody surgery can be and how raucous the process is, with music played by many doctors, and banter and cross-talk among the staff.

When I walked into my first operation, I was surprised to see the entire patient covered with the sterile sheets known as surgical drapes. Only the relatively small area that comprised the surgical field—the part of the body on which surgeons were operating—was exposed. With the patient's face, arms, and legs all blocked from view, I found it remarkably easy to forget that this procedure involved an actual human being, especially since the only people monitoring the patient's responses were the anesthesiologist and his or her nurses. During my first few surgeries, I was periodically startled out of my concentration on the procedure whenever the surgeon asked the anesthesiologist, "How's our patient doing?"

The most surprising aspect of my first surgery was the smell of burning flesh. This particular surgeon cut into his patient with a scalpel, then immediately burned the bleeding edges of the wound with a tiny cauterizing tool. Over the years, I've tried to describe the smell of burning flesh and the closest I can come is freshly burned toast thrown into a skillet already simmering with rotten fish, pork fat, and an old leather shoe. However, even that description may not do justice to the aroma. All I can say is that anyone who has ever experienced it recognizes it instantly. It's not like the smell of a fresh steak slapped on a grill: The odor of roasting *human* flesh is nauseating, pure and simple. And the sound of that cautery knife was horrible. I had to stop myself from jumping each time the surgeon touched it to the patient's flesh. Every time the knife hit the end of a bleeding blood vessel, I heard a little *ssst,* like the sound when you put a match into water. *Ssst . . .* and a fresh burst of the smell . . . a tiny tendril of smoke, rising into the air.

As the surgery proceeded, I was especially struck by the smell of warm blood that pervaded the room. The smells of surgery are something the medical shows haven't conveyed at all. While burning human flesh smells nothing like its animal counterpart, human and animal blood smell eerily the same—and as someone who had done her share of hunting and butchering wild game, I hadn't expected the smell of blood to bother me. But it did, maybe because of the visuals that went with it. Every so often, the surgeon would hit an artery and blood would spew up like a tiny geyser. Even the smallest artery could cause an arc of blood to splat across his blue-green robe.

Although I loved watching these surgeries, I realized early on that I'd never make it as a pathologist. Frankly, I don't like to see or smell blood. I can't stand to see someone insert a needle into an eyeball to withdraw fluid, and the sounds and smells associated with aspirating stomach contents make me want to vomit up mine. Even today, I avoid the "squishy stuff" whenever possible and I'm profoundly grateful that

I was able to go into first orthopedics and then forensic anthropology, where I could work with muscle and bone rather than internal organs.

Nevertheless, my class in pathology, where we, shoulder to shoulder with the medical students, would watch pathologists perform autopsies, gave me a valuable insight into my own capacities. My budding ability to visualize a body in three dimensions began to pay off: Before the pathologist made the first cut through the skin, I knew precisely what he or she would find underneath. Since I now knew what normal organs and tissue should look like, abnormalities caused by disease or injury seemed glaringly obvious.

It's one thing to stand at a surgeon's elbow and watch the most intricate procedures. It's a whole other thing to perform surgery yourself. The Medical College of Georgia believed that in order to illustrate surgery properly, medical illustrators had to pick up the knife and know how to use it. Of course, we illustrators were never going to operate on our own patients. But if we had never performed operations ourselves, how would we discover how much tension is needed to suture intestines, and how that differs from suturing skin? How would we learn exactly how to hold each instrument, or the correct direction and technique for applying force when retracting a rib cage? And if we didn't thoroughly understand these procedures, how could we translate such information to our drawings? These were things we could only learn by doing.

So in its wisdom, the Medical College had decided that we illustrators would enroll alongside the budding surgeons in their classes in dog surgery. Each of us students—future doctors and illustrators alike— were assigned a large dog who'd been abandoned or donated to our program, on whom we could learn the basics of surgical technique.

From the first, I had mixed feelings about this aspect of our training. On one hand, I love dogs—always do, always have. So I wasn't without sympathy for the critics of the Georgia program, who considered it cruel, disgusting, even unethical for us illustration students to cut up helpless animals in order to learn surgical techniques that we were never going to perform.

On the other hand, the dog surgery program turned out to be one of the most valuable experiences in my education. Here was where I really began to understand what surgeons experienced—because, albeit it on a very small scale, I was doing their work. Each dog in the program received a thorough medical "workup," then underwent a series of operations over a period of several weeks. We removed their gall bladders and spleens, and resectioned their bowels. Working around the clock, we did everything we could to ease their post-op pain. All of us, illustrators and med students alike, were deeply committed to our dogs' care.

The most surprising thing to me about actually performing surgery for the first time was that the tissue I was operating on was *warm*. The only tissue I'd ever handled before had been in the dissection lab, and it was almost icy. Now suddenly my hands were warmed with the vital heat of a living creature, a warmth that crept up through my fingers and wrists and into my arms. It wasn't unpleasant, exactly, but it was a shock.

Being a dog lover, I had bonded with my dog patient as I performed the series of operations on him. He was a large German shepherd with melting brown eyes, and I never failed to spend a few minutes on each "medical" visit scratching him behind the ears and telling him how beautiful he was. Although I purposely never gave him a name, I did manage to block out the fact that our final exam required us to euthanize our dogs and perform autopsies on them.

For the medical students, this was a crucial rite of passage: Could they maintain the detachment they would need to cut open human bodies, to depersonalize their patients enough to be able to work on them? We illustrators felt that we were entitled to a bit more artistic sensitivity—but, truthfully, the process was hard on all of us. We tried to rationalize it, saying that if these dogs hadn't been part of our program, they would have been killed anyway.

That argument was fine in theory, but when I actually had to approach my dog's cage, look into his eyes, and contemplate ending his life, I knew I simply couldn't do it. I went to my professor and begged for a dispensation. He looked into my face for what seemed like several minutes and I couldn't help wondering what he was thinking. "Fine," he said at last. "You don't have to be there when the animal dies."

I still had to perform the autopsy, but at least I didn't have to perform that awful act. Looking back, I realize this was an important turning point for me. I had no problem with dead bodies, but I couldn't handle the process of dying. Wherever I worked as a medical illustrator, it wouldn't be in a hospital.

Now I understand that the dog surgery class was important for another reason: It was crucial preparation for the forensic cases I'd later encounter in which the stories of the victims were absolutely heartrending—children led into certain death by their trusted parents, as happened with the Branch Davidians in Waco, Texas; a battered wife and murdered infants shot in cold blood by a Kentucky father; the young woman butchered and thrown into the chilly Wisconsin River. What I started to learn in dog surgery—and have had to relearn many times since—is the crucial balance between becoming hardened enough to remain objective with the science while retaining enough emotion to feel outrage on the victims' behalf. Cold, clear objectivity enables me to analyze the evidence, and that's a crucial part of my job, one that offers closure to loved ones and sometimes helps bring a murderer to justice. But compassion for the victim spurs me on to uncover new evidence, keeping me up late to work on a forensic sculpture or sending me on another trip into the Kentucky woods. It's so frustrating when my colleagues and I can't identify a victim or find the crucial evidence in his or her case—but it's so rewarding when we can.

•　　•　　•

My experience with dog surgery had taught me that I couldn't work in a hospital—but then where could I practice my profession? Through a series of fortunate coincidences, my ongoing interest in muscles and bones led me to Jack Hughston, M.D., who was then doing groundbreaking work in orthopedics and sports medicine at the Hughston Orthopaedic Clinic in Columbus, Georgia. To my eternal gratitude, Dr. Hughston not only hired me, but also gave me numerous opportunities to expand my knowledge of anatomy, orthopedics, and illustration, and over the next fifteen years I made thousands of drawings based on anatomical dissections and surgeries conducted at the clinic. I was even able to conduct dissections of my own, working with hundreds of knees, ankles, hips, shoulders, and elbows—extremities from men and women of all races and ages. Here, in the clinic's sterile, cold, and often lonely lab, I began to think of myself as teasing secrets from the dead, forever grateful that their final gift would help others regain the function of an injured or diseased limb.

For several years, my participation at the clinic was deeply satisfying. Eventually, though, I felt that I'd come to a standstill. My drawing skills couldn't keep up with my advancement as an anatomist: I was now at the point where I could see things that I couldn't draw. I simply couldn't make my hands reproduce on paper what I could perceive on the cadaver specimen—but my sculpting skills, I thought, were somewhat better. So, almost on a whim, I decided to create three-dimensional wax sculptures to portray the anatomical details I knew were there. Ironically, I'd always enjoyed sculpture more than work in two dimensions; but, until now, I'd had no outlet for this skill.

But when I approached Dr. Hughston, full of enthusiasm for my new idea, I was a bit taken aback by his response. "Sculptures? Clay models? We're not running an art gallery here, Emily. This is a clinic, in case you've forgotten."

Eventually, I won Dr. Hughston's permission to work on the sculptures in the lab—but on my own time. All of a sudden, I was leading a double life. Every day, I would put in my usual full day's work producing drawings. Every evening, I would labor for hours sculpting life-sized clay models of knees in various stages of dissection, going far past the usual details portrayed in medical textbooks to reveal the pioneering discoveries that Dr. Hughston and his colleagues had made. His anatomical research revealed intricate fibers in the knee, shoulder, and ankle that had never before been shown by medical illustrators—until now.

To ensure accuracy, I brought specimens of fresh amputations right into my art studio. With my left hand, I felt my way along the joint, sometimes staring at the structures, sometimes closing my eyes and trying to send some secret code to my brain. I concentrated my entire being on what my hand was feeling—the contours of the knee, its bumps and curves, the spots where it was soft and spongy, the places where it was hard and smooth. Then, with my right hand, I rendered what I felt into the soft, oily clay. Although I could never have completed this project without a detailed knowledge of anatomy, working on this sculpture was a true leap into the unknown for me, combining science, art, and intuition in my first attempt to make a model come alive.

When my first sculpture was finished, I couldn't wait to show it to Dr. Hughston. He was more taciturn than usual as I ushered him into my studio. But when I lifted the soft cloth to uncover my wax model of a human knee, he was dumbfounded. Pioneer that he was, he saw the possibilities at once.

"Well," he said after a long pause, in which I eagerly sought to read his blank expression. "Looks like I was wrong. We sure can make use of this."

With Dr. Hughston's enthusiastic support, I went on to create over two dozen wax models of knees, shoulders, and ankles, pictures of which are still in use today. My work set a new international standard for medical education, creating a reputation for me as well as for the clinic. Yet though I seemed to be at the top of my profession, I realized that I had never really become the scientist I had always wanted to be. I had loved making drawings and sculptures—but they were always in service of a doctor or surgeon's work. I wanted a chance to do my own work with the human body, to take the lead in research and investigation instead of forever following two steps behind.

Medical illustration seemed to be running out of challenges—but I was still intrigued by the prospect of learning how to do a facial reconstruction for the West Point murder case. So off I went to Betty Pat's weeklong seminar in Norman, Oklahoma—where I was immediately sucked into the fascination of forensic work.

We started with the principles behind the different facial tissue depths. Think of a human face—what determines its shapes and contours? Most of it, of course, is bone structure. But the differing soft tissues are what turn the skull into a unique face that we recognize as male or female, Black or White, old or young. Scientists have developed a complex series of mathematical formulas giving the basic information on how sex, race, and other factors help to create different-shaped skulls and different patterns of tissue depth and shape.

To start a sculpture, then, we learned how to use these formulas to cut small erasers into different lengths and glue them on to the skull, to approximate the skin depths at various key points. Then we learned how to "connect the dots" by covering the erasers with clay, building up the contours that mimicked a real human face.

This would be challenging enough if our only goal were to produce a lifelike image. But ultimately, we wanted to create a face that resembled a specific person—a person whom we had never seen. Somehow we had to envision the victim's face and re-create something close to it, so that someone who had known this person could recognize him or her and come forward with a name.

During Betty Pat's weeklong class, I listened in awe to more stories of my teacher's most interesting cases. Then, at night, she and the instructors in the composite drawing class—conducted right next door to our reconstruction class—would discuss the profession of forensic art. As far as I could see, medical and forensic art were fairly similar. The primary difference seemed to be in the payoff. As a medical illustrator, I felt a certain satisfaction in a job well done and the knowledge that I was helping to teach anatomy and surgery to physicians. But that pleasure paled beside the thrill of being part of a team that solved murder mysteries and helped bring killers to justice.

Back I went to the Hughston Clinic, totally hooked on facial reconstruction. Although I was still nervous about doing the sculpture that

Brian's colleagues had requested, I was now eager to try. However, the skills that had seemed so temptingly within my reach in Betty Pat's class appeared maddeningly elusive now. Like so many people, I initially thought that facial reconstruction could be reduced to a formula or recipe. If you followed the recipe, you would get a good result. Boy, was I wrong! Sure, you had to know the basics, but then there was all kinds of room for judgment—and for error.

Good student that I was, I followed the recipe I'd learned from Betty Pat. I checked out the formula for a White male, cut the appropriate markers, and glued them on to the skull. Then, to the best of my ability, I covered everything with clay, sculpting eyelids, mouth, and nose to correspond to the bony structure of the underlying bones and teeth. The final result did somewhat resemble a man's face, but to me it was an extreme caricature. The eyes were buggy, the mouth looked like it belonged on a puppet, and I didn't yet understand how important the neck was to make a person look "real."

None of the cops had any evidence of individualizing details that might make this man's face unique. Did he have a moustache? A beard? Did he wear eyeglasses? Was he bald? Nobody knew—and that made it more difficult.

Although the police were relatively happy with my work, I was not. My frustration led me to what turned out to be a groundbreaking idea. Before I'd left for Betty Pat's class, I'd been working on new computer graphic techniques for demonstrating surgical procedures. I now had the idea of using computer graphics to produce what I called a "postmortem lineup." By using the computer to apply facial hair, eyeglasses, and several different hairstyles to a single clay sculpture, I gave a range of different looks to that same face.

The completed facial reconstruction might not have been a striking success, but the first-time use of a computer-enhanced postmortem lineup sent a sensational wave through the law enforcement community. When we publicized the case in the Columbus newspaper, trying to identify the victim, the reporter was more astounded with the computer enhancements and variations than with the actual case. Forensic artists across the country quickly adopted my technique for computer-enhanced facial reconstruction, and, with some modifications, it is still in use today. Although my initial foray into the field never produced a victim ID, it seemed I had made a contribution nonetheless.

•   •   •

It would take me three years of trial and error before I felt I had mastered computer-enhanced facial reconstruction. Still, because I was the only person in the Alabama, Georgia, and North Florida region doing this kind of work, the local police knew me and they starting bringing me all their toughest cases—the ones they just couldn't ID on their own, cases that had gone unsolved for months and even years. Once again, I was working at the clinic all day and leading a secret life at night. And, once again, I was becoming frustrated with my skills as an artist. Give me a bone, a ligament, or a muscle and I'll draw you up a beauty, but when it comes to the human face, you might want to get yourself another illustrator. I was an expert at drawing internal organs, but I couldn't draw faces—I wasn't a portrait artist.

My work with law enforcement was satisfying, though, and I reveled in my newfound camaraderie with police and prosecutors. The more I enjoyed forensic work, the less able I became to put aside my frustrations with the Hughston Clinic. Meanwhile, my experimental computer-assisted techniques had made a modest splash in the law enforcement community, and, along with Karen Burns, I was invited to present them at the July 1990 annual meeting of the International Association for Identification (IAI) in Nashville, Tennessee. Like so many other serendipitous events in my life, this one was to prove a turning point.

I arrived at the conference full of anticipation, thrilled to meet so many forensic artists as well as investigators, forensic scientists, and others in the law enforcement field—people of substance and commitment, dedicated to a cause larger than themselves. These were people I really respected, people with whom I'd be proud to work.

My own presentation went well, and for that I was grateful. My new buddies offered their congratulations. Then they told me that the one presentation I must not miss was the one on forensic anthropology at the "Body Farm"—the world-famous department of forensic anthropology at the University of Tennessee at Knoxville, where bodies were literally left to rot on the ground so students and professors could observe and measure the process of decomposition.

This was years before Patricia Cornwell's novel about the place was published. I'd heard about the Body Farm in Betty Pat's workshop, though I confess I hadn't thought much about it. Now, though, I went to the talk by Knoxville doctoral student Murray Marks (who later became one of the nation's foremost professors of forensic anthropology). From the moment that Murray began speaking, I was riveted. And when he speculated on the development of computer technology that could "someday" be used to aid in victim identification, I sat bolt upright in my seat. WHAT!!! You mean I was already on the right track? Anthropology Ph.D.s were just now thinking about this?

That was it. I knew what I wanted to do and where I wanted to do it. I rushed up to Murray after his lecture and excitedly told him what I had been doing on my own to develop the method he'd said was still "pie in the sky." He was impressed, and urged me to come to Knoxville to apply for one of the coveted slots as a Ph.D. student under Dr. Bill Bass.

I was powerfully drawn to the world of forensic anthropology that Murray described to me that day. But I was now forty-three years old and at the peak of my current profession. Did I really have the strength to start over?

Then came the case of "Baby Lollipops."

In the fall of 1990, four months after the conference, Detective Charlie Metscher of the Miami Beach Police Department called for my help in identifying a three-year-old child whose emaciated and battered remains had been found under shrubs in a residential area just a few days earlier. Police and medical examiners surmised that the child had likely lain there alive but unable to move as his brain swelled, he became dehydrated, and his life slowly slipped away. In addition to numerous acute cuts and bruises, he was suffering from a recent head fracture, a brain injury, and a massive hemorrhage that involved his left leg and hip. Older injuries covered his entire body, with broken bones in so many stages of healing that it was almost impossible to count the number of times he had been beaten. This child had not only been abused—tortured really—but he had also been starved. Apparently close to three years old, he had weighed only eighteen pounds when he died. Because the tiny T-shirt he had been wearing had a pattern of large lollipops across the chest, the press had dubbed him "Baby Lollipops."

The discovery of this child and the revelation of the horrors he had endured united the Miami community in a common fury. But the investigation couldn't proceed until the police knew who the child was. Because the crime had been so brutal, the media and police agreed that photos of the child's battered, bruised, and swollen body should not be made public. Nevertheless, he needed a face.

As it happened, Detective Metscher had been in the audience at my presentation in Nashville. He wanted me to use my techniques to create an image of Baby Lollipops that could be circulated throughout South Florida.

Of course I said yes. I was as outraged as he was over the case, and I was determined to do everything in my power to help solve it.

A child dead from abuse evokes a very deep reaction in even the most hardened professionals. The seemingly never-ending litany of tiny bodies with ulcerated burns, torn-off fingers and toes, or huge foreign objects forced into their rectums and vaginas cries out for justice or retribution or both. No professional, no matter how accomplished, ever gets used to the kinds of horrors that we see on a daily basis—we don't become inured to the terrible things that people can do to each other. We do, however, fall into a routine. It may take something truly terrible to shock us. Cops who hide their emotions with cynicism and jokes revert back to human beings again when faced with a victim like Baby Lollipops.

There was also a sense of urgency: Charlie Metscher and I both knew that time was of the essence. Now that the child had been found, there was a good chance that the perpetrators would skip town and never be seen again.

Charlie immediately sent me the photo of the boy and a scenario of the case. I became obsessed with my mission and stayed up two nights in a row, experimenting with as-yet-untested methods that combined photography, digitized images, and computer graphics.

My own limits as a portrait artist had, some months before, pushed me to modify another technique that was now being used by forensic artists doing composite drawings to nab suspects. I called it "facial restoration." I began by photographing victims' faces that, for various reasons, couldn't be used for public viewing, digitized the images, and then used the computer to cut out the eyes, noses, and mouths. Then, from my homemade computerized file of facial features, I selected features that I thought would most closely resemble those of my victim. I inserted these "new" facial features into the victim's picture and then blended the whole portrait until it appeared as one "natural" face, a sort of computer-assisted "Mr. Potato Head."

Since most of Baby Lollipops's flesh was still intact, I could smooth out the skin's defects with computerized airbrushing. The software program enabled me to draw new lips over the cut and bruised lips in the picture, even as I maintained the integrity of their original size and general shape. I was feeling optimistic about rendering a convincing image when I ran into a new problem: the eyes.

In the photograph, Baby Lollipops's eyes had been swollen shut, but I wanted to show him with normal, healthy, open eyes. Yet try as I might, I couldn't make the eyes look right when I drew them on the computer. I tried drawing the eyes on a separate sheet of paper and then downloading them into my image, but there was too great a gap between my drawing and the photographed face.

So I turned to one of my colleagues at the clinic for help. By now, people at work knew all about my "secret life," and they had all been very supportive, even to the point of letting me videotape their faces to create the computerized file of features I used in my clay facial-reconstruction experiments. But when I tried to use these same cutout facial features on Baby Lollipops, I ran into a few unexpected problems. First, my fledgling technique had been designed for use with straight-on photos, whereas the crime scene photos of the battered child had been taken at an angle. And, of course, there were no infant faces in the computer "library" I had created. I asked one of my friends to let me digitize her child's face, and when I sat the little boy down in my studio, I turned the camera ever so slightly, trying to match the angle of the little boy in the autopsy photograph. Back at the computer, I left the image of the T-shirt and the child's shoulders just as they were, but I inserted these new eyes into the face I had restored. I only needed the eyes, because with the computer I had already smoothed over the bruised and decomposed features of Baby Lollipops's face.

Finally, instead of letting the image look like a photograph of a real dead child with a new nose, eyes, and lips, I blended and airbrushed the entire face and head so that it all looked like a drawing of a live little boy. His eyes were open, his lips were closed, and I purposely arched the eyebrows just the tiniest bit to make it appear as if the boy were puzzled—or pleading.

The visual effect was powerful, and when the coroner and detectives released their autopsy information, the poignantly illustrated story made the front page of most major newspapers in Florida, as well as the TV show *America's Most Wanted*. Although there would normally be a stigma associated with releasing a photograph of a dead infant to the media, the fact that my image looked so alive enabled both police and press to use the picture with a clear conscience.

Although I was anguished over the case of this battered child, I confess I also felt a kind of exhilaration. For the first time in my life, I was a real member of the forensic team. Before I'd always been "Brian's girlfriend" or "that artist from the clinic," and the law enforcement personnel treated me with the kind of politeness reserved for outsiders. This time I was a member of the team, first and foremost, and my colleagues on the force weren't afraid to show me their desperation, to share their hopes, fears, and frustration. Nor were they intimidated by the fact that I happened to have a skill that they lacked. Unlike a few of the doctors I'd been working with for the past fifteen years, these guys were far too confident of their own abilities to even think of being threatened by mine.

Then there was the elation of knowing that I'd helped with a case that cried out for justice. Soon after my picture of Baby Lollipops was published, the police were deluged with calls, and by early December they found and arrested the child's mother, Ana Maria Cardona, and her lover, Olivia Gonzalez. A suspicious babysitter had come forward on her own, the day before my picture had even reached the airwaves. She was initially able to tentatively identify Baby Lollipops as Lazaro Figueroa from his description—but she wasn't absolutely certain until she saw my picture.

That picture galvanized both her resolve and the community as a whole. Lazaro had essentially been invisible throughout his short, miserable life. Testimony at trial confirmed that he had spent most of his days tied to a post inside a closet. There were no pictures of him anywhere in existence. But once he had a face, the investigation really came alive. People who knew about Lazaro were finally willing to cooperate with detectives, feeding them the information that enabled them to locate and arrest his mother.

My picture had energized both the cops and the community. And as investigators looked for information about Lazaro's life, they also uncovered several new cases of child abuse. Apparently, people saw the picture and started calling to check on all the other little kids they knew. They also forced friends, family, and welfare officials to check on potentially at-risk children.

Eventually, Gonzalez cut a deal and agreed to testify in exchange for a sentence that would spare her life. At Lazaro's mother's trial, Gonzalez's gripping testimony revealed that the boy had been beaten repeatedly with broomsticks, belts, and finally with a baseball bat. Testimony also revealed that the boy's mother would also intentionally poke his eyes, break dinner plates over his head, and smear his face with his own feces. As a result of Gonzalez's testimony, Ana Maria Cardona was found guilty and eventually sentenced to death in Florida's electric chair (although the verdict was vacated in July 2002).

The case of Baby Lollipops changed my life. For the first time, I had gotten personally involved with a gripping, heart-wrenching case. For the first time, I was on the inside. And when the whole investigation came together and they got a conviction, *what a rush!* I had never felt anything like it in my life.

So as the Baby Lollipops case concluded, my soul-searching did, too. I applied for one of the few grad-student slots at the University of Tennessee at Knoxville. In December, I gave my six months' notice to the clinic. In May, I packed my bags and left.

"Remember," said Dr. Hughston as I started to pull out of his driveway on my way to Knoxville, "you can always come back." He reached in through the window and put that big loving hand on my shoulder, giving it a little shake, just to let me know he meant what he said. Whatever the future held, I knew I was on my way and that I had my mentor's approval. I waved goodbye to Dr. Hughston and Columbus, and headed off to the Body Farm.

2

Death and Decay

In nature nothing dies. From each sad remnant of decay,
some forms of life arise . . .
— C H A R L E S   M A C K A Y

The FIRST THING I noticed was the smell—a sweet, almost musty odor, such a subtle part of the light spring breeze ruffling our hair that I couldn't quite tell where it came from.

I was following closely in the footsteps of Murray Marks, the guide on my first trip to the infamous Body Farm. This was always the first rite of passage for any grad student in the forensic anthropology program—a trip out to the small field and hardwood forest behind the University of Tennessee Medical Center in Knoxville.

Suddenly, Murray stopped and nodded toward the ground at my feet. Murray was tall and handsome, with dark-brown hair and soulful brown eyes, and I was happy to follow his gaze, but I could see only a black stain hidden in the tall grass. No, wait, there was more. If I looked closely at the mucky matrix of soil, dead foliage, and thousands of small brown pellets, I could see something else—the barely discernable bones of a human forearm.

I did everything I could to keep my face composed, though I'm sure I didn't fool Murray for a second. This skeleton was different from any I had seen in my medical career. The bones seemed to have soaked up the wetness and color of the soil, with bits of dark gray-brown sinew clinging to their ends in a futile attempt to hold them together at the joints. Where the larger joints had not yet come apart it looked as though someone had frozen a Halloween skeleton marionette in the middle of a wild dance: the legs splayed at the knees, one foot turned in as the other stuck straight up with curled toes, one arm folded awkwardly behind the neck while the other reached for something far off in the grass. The skull was there, but it appeared to be on backwards— the face was hidden in the dirt, while the jawbone rested at a strange angle within the chest cavity.

"How long do you think that body's been here?" Murray asked.

I looked again. Until today, I had only known bones as part of a whole, linked by the wires that keep a laboratory teaching skeleton intact, or as a dynamic living framework connected by ligaments. After death, though, those tissues begin to decay, and soon there is quite literally nothing to hold the bones together. Now I could see that when a corpse is laid out on the ground, gravity sucks the bones downward so that the skeleton eventually collapses, settling into earth made soft and soggy from the decaying tissues. What once was a rib cage becomes a flat row of rib bones, while the spine turns into a collection of disarticulated vertebrae. Of course, the skull and jawbone— mandible, to use the technical term—are easy to spot, but the tiny ligaments that hold our teeth in place also go the way of all flesh. Unless the root's shape keeps it stuck inside the socket, the teeth fall out, too.

"How long has it been here?" Murray repeated.

I took a closer look. The two forearm bones—the radius and ulna— had come completely detached from each other, and there wasn't a single bit of flesh on either the hand bones or the skull. "Six months?" I guessed.

Murray laughed.

"Nine months?" I ventured. "A year?"

He laughed again. "Two weeks," he told me.

"Two weeks?"

"Because of the maggots."

"The *what*?" I looked more closely at the mushy ground and took an involuntary step backward. I hadn't noticed them at first, though I had been puzzled by the shiny little dark-brown shells littering the ground at my feet, but now I saw that all around the periphery of the skeleton were dozens of milky-white, slow-moving maggots, bucking like inchworms, on their way to some unknown destination.

Later I would learn that these little creatures have helped solved many murders. Now, though, I was blissfully unaware that those maggots were a huge part of what lay in store for me as a forensic anthropologist. Murray watched with amusement as I tried to lean closer to see the skull without letting the toes of my brand-new running shoes actually touch anything that seemed even faintly maggot-related.

As Murray and I left the decaying human remains, he explained to me a little of the Body Farm's history. In the early 1970s, the program's chair, Dr. William Bass, ran into a roadblock as he tried to solve a case involving a decomposed body. His interest in the process of human decay was piqued when he realized that, amazingly, no one had ever studied this process before, despite its obvious usefulness in forensic investigation. He also knew that U.T. Knoxville didn't have a modern skeletal collection for him to teach osteology or to use as a forensic anthropology database. The school did have a good collection of bones from Native American archaeological sites, but these were too different in size and shape to be of much use in current forensic research.

So Bass asked the University of Tennessee to give him a small section of land where he could leave human bodies to decompose under natural conditions and then gather the bones for his collection. After all, nature's method of stripping a carcass is fast and efficient, and it doesn't cost a cent. People who had donated their bodies to science found their way onto the Body Farm; so did unidentified and unclaimed corpses from the local medical examiner. Nature did its work—and Dr. Bass and his graduate students were able to document the processes by which bodies decay.

Until Dr. Bass came along, forensic scientists who were asked to establish time since death of a badly decomposed or skeletonized body had to rely upon guesswork and experience, laboriously comparing each new case with earlier solved cases. Now, thanks to Dr. Bass's pioneering work, we have documented scientific studies to back up our hunches. Despite the obvious advantages to this method of study, the University of Tennessee at Knoxville is still the only place in the world where scientists can observe and document the day-to-day journey from death to skeletonization.

Now, as Murray and I walked out from the woods full of corpses into the open field, I saw his look of approval. I hadn't fainted or gasped in horror—on the contrary, I'd been fascinated, drawing nearer for a closer look, even asking an intelligent question or two. All things considered, I'd approached the dead body like a scientist rather than a voyeur—and I realized that I had passed a test. True, I'd seen Murray's slides and heard his descriptions at his lecture the summer before. But I had to admit, seeing the real thing was something else.

As Murray steered me over to two white cars and opened the trunks to see how the newest body-decay project was going, I couldn't help feeling just a bit triumphant. I knew that Dr. Bass had insisted that I—like all other incoming grad students—be taken out to the decay facility as soon as possible. If I wasn't prepared to deal with decomposing bodies—and with all other aspects of death and decay—it was best to find out now. Well, so far so good. But what other tests were in store for me?

·   ·   ·

I soon found out. Within only a few weeks, I was told to design and carry out a short-term research project of my own. Since I'd come to the university with an avid interest in facial reconstruction, I thought it would be interesting to document the changes in a person's face as he or she decayed. While still in Georgia, I'd been asked to "restore" faces that were in various stages of decomposition and I'd had some success, both with traditional drawing techniques and with experimental computer enhancement. In my naïveté, I thought that once I established some predictable baseline parameters for facial decomposition, all I'd have to do was take a photo of a dead person's face and perform a simple computer maneuver to make him or her look alive again.

I was wrong. Okay, I was right in theory—but only if I got to the body within the first day and a half. After that, if it was warm and humid enough, the maggots would have done their work and the face would be irrevocably altered, making any photos totally useless for identification purposes.

However, I was still interested in documenting what happened as maggots destroyed a face and, as luck would have it, I got my chance the very next day, when a newly donated body arrived at our lab just hours after the man had died. I positioned the man carefully on his back out in the open field, not too far from the wooded area. Securing his head with a rock on either side, I spread the camera tripod right over his shoulders and pointed the lens down toward his face at a ninety-degree angle. To my satisfaction, I was able to get a shot in before the first fly had landed.

For the next four days and nights, I returned to the body, remounted the camera, and took a new picture—every four hours. I scaled back to every six hours for the next ten days after that. May in Tennessee is indeed hot and humid, so the flies had laid their eggs the same day I put the body there, and by the next afternoon, the man's nose and mouth were bulging with baby maggots and fly eggs. In the middle of the following night, under the stark beam of my flashlight, his lips seemed to move as if he were trying to speak—I even thought I heard him moaning. No, those sounds were mine, involuntary responses to the sight of what had once been a human face being devoured from the inside out.

It took everything I had to focus the camera and zoom in on the maggot masses that were churning inside this man's mouth and nose and under his eyelids, creating this roiling, seething motion as they fed. Lines of ants were streaming up from the ground, ready to devour any maggots unlucky enough to be pushed out toward the edge of the teeming mass. It was a little unnerving to realize that however much we like to think we're at the top of the food chain while we're alive, once we're dead, we're just part of it.

After I left the facility that night, I went home and quickly poured a therapeutic dose of bourbon over a few ice cubes. As I sat on my back porch, drinking slowly and trying to regain some composure, I seriously doubted if I was cut out for this kind of work.

I managed to sleep for a few hours, but my dreams were filled with crawling maggots and voracious ants. At dawn, back at the facility, two startled vultures who had been trying to disembowel a nearby body flew to the trees directly over my head. As they took off slowly and clumsily from their breakfast, they followed their usual practice of spewing vomit on rapid takeoff—vomit that fell at my feet and over my corpse's torso. Meanwhile, slimy trails of the snails who had visited the carcass during the predawn hours now crisscrossed my subject's face, and his cheeks spewed adolescent maggots who seemed to be growing bigger right before my eyes. Maggots were pouring from his nostrils, too, and they had almost finished snacking on the last traces of his eyeballs, leaving empty sockets in his skull. Stifling a sigh, I forced myself to step over this man's body and set up my tripod.

·   ·   ·

Entomologists analyze maggots, adult flies, other insects, and similar small scavengers to estimate when and where a person died, and to help determine the types of injuries a victim has suffered. Adult flies— the very same houseflies that buzz around your picnic dinner—can sense death immediately. They are drawn to a body within a few minutes of when death occurs and, if they have access to the carcass, they land and start surveying the territory. Appearances to the contrary, when they crawl around on the body, they aren't eating much—just looking for the ideal place to lay their eggs. The tiny eggs, which resemble little clumps of sawdust, hatch into maggots within a day or two. The maggots immediately start to devour the carcass, growing visibly bigger with each passing day.

At first they don't even resemble the fat, stubby little legless larvae with soft white skin that most people visualize when they hear the word. Maggots have to go through three developmental stages, or "instars." Their pale, white, papery skin splits and they shed it each time, until finally these mobile, voracious little eating machines have passed from infancy through their teenage days to reach their full growth potential.

Then, when they just can't eat any more, they crawl away from the dead body to find a place to hide. Their soft white skin becomes a dark-brown pupa casing, or shell, shaped something like a miniature football about one-fourth to one-half inch long, within which they metamorphose into adult flies—much as a caterpillar changes into a butterfly within a cocoon. If the weather stays warm and humid, the adult fly breaks open the end of its shell after a week or two, and the cycle is complete. At that point, if by any chance there's anything left of the body, the cycle begins again—and then again. If the entomologist can calculate the cycle, he or she can help you estimate when the dead body was first exposed to the elements.

Time of death is just one of the factors an entomologist helps to determine. Since the insects and other arthropods (spiders, mites, centipedes) commonly found on bodies have preferred habitats, sometimes an entomologist can tell if a person was moved after he or she was killed. If a corpse found in Florida is colonized by a species found only in New Jersey and parts north, the authorities are likely to include the possibility that the body was brought in from someplace else.

Sometimes maggots can even help you figure out whether a person sustained any injuries at the time of death. When the adult flies lay their eggs, they seek out the sites that provide the best environment for their young. In the human body, that would be the mouth, nose, ears, eyes, and genitals—warm, moist, and dark. The flies burrow as far as they can into those tempting, secret places and lay their eggs. In a decaying corpse, therefore, you would expect to see early maggot concentrations there—and if they've congregated anywhere else, perhaps another body part was broken or bloody at the time of death.

What still amazes me is how quickly maggots can reduce a fleshy corpse to bone. That childhood rhyme of "The worms crawl in, the worms crawl out" is not far wrong. There's a saying among forensic entomologists: Three flies and their offspring can consume a carcass as quickly as can a full-grown lion. Not bad for tiny creatures less than an inch long.

By the time I finished my time-lapse portrayal of decay, I was no longer fazed by sights—and smells—that two weeks ago had left me nauseated and trembling. Somehow, the shocking had become commonplace, and the human remains I saw rotting in the sun had begun to look more like three-dimensional puzzles and less like once-living beings. As I would later learn, this kind of detachment had its price— but it was also the necessary precondition for doing this work. If I was ever to learn to estimate the postmortem interval—how long it had been since someone had died—or to read the story of a person's last hours in a few broken bones, I would have to look at human remains as though I were a disembodied representative of science, not as a woman whose own body would one day end up rotting in the ground like everybody else's.

I still don't like maggots, though. Never have. Never will.

•   •   •

"I have a new challenge for you, class," said Dr. Bass. On his desk he placed a metal cafeteria-style tray filled with a collection of human bones.

"I must confess," he went on, "I don't have high hopes. In twenty years, no one has ever gotten this one right."

I'd just finished a semester of Bill Bass's osteology class, where he'd done his best to initiate me and a dozen other grad students into the science of bone. Now we were taking the next giant step into the mysteries of forensic anthropology.

Forensic anthropologists take what we as physical anthropologists have learned about bone and apply it to criminal investigations. In the ideal world, physical anthropologists can look at a skeleton and tell you several basic pieces of information: age, race, sex, and stature. They can probably also tell you something about bone diseases and trauma—broken bones, healed injuries, and other evidence of how the person may have lived or died.

Of course, most anthropologists are usually working with centuries-old skeletons. We forensic anthropologists do the same kind of work—but on people who may have died only a few years, months, or even days ago. Our work may also involve fresh but unassociated body parts—the kind normally encountered in high-impact plane crashes or explosions—as well as corpses partially destroyed by fire.

As part of our academic training, my classmates and I were required to study cultural anthropology and theory of archaeology, and I'd struggled mightily through those classes. But I got my reward when it was finally time to learn about bone. No two ways about it, bone fascinated me.

True, Dr. Bass was an incredibly demanding professor, which I must admit I resented at first, particularly since, at Dr. Hughston's clinic, I'd been considered something of a bone expert myself. I soon came to find out, though, that it wasn't the same at all. The bones at the clinic might be broken or even crushed—but they were always safely encased within a recognizable portion of the human anatomy, always connected to their neighboring bones just as nature intended. As a forensic anthropologist, I would not always have the luxury of whole bones. A murderer might deliberately shatter his victims' bones, or a dog, bear, or coyote might crunch the bones between its teeth. And fire could reduce a human skeleton to mere fragments with devastating efficiency.

As a result, Dr. Bass insisted that we be able to instantly identify small fragments of bone, as well as the whole bones that are standard fare in most anatomy and anthropology classes. This seemed like a daunting challenge at first, but we soon learned that all bones have identifying features that make them unique, distinguishing each bone from every other and even separating right from left. For example, the metacarpals—the bones extending from the palm of the hand—all look alike at first glance, but if you look at the end that joins the wrist bones, you can see that each has a slightly different shape.

Once we'd learned the secrets of each individual bone, we had to be able to look at a fragment and pick out the one feature that would help us identify it. The mandibular condyle, for instance, is a tiny part of the jawbone that fits into the corresponding groove of the skull—no bigger than a plump raisin. It has a shape that is unlike any other piece of the human skeleton, and once its image is firmly anchored in your mind, you can not only recognize it, you can tell which side of the jaw it comes from, even if the rest of the jaw is missing.

As soon as we started to feel the first glimmer of confidence in our ability to identify adult skeletal material, we had to step back in time and learn how these bones looked while they were still growing. The bones of newborns and infants were a wonder to behold, but the differences in shape and size from adult bones added yet another element of confusion. Soon I learned, though, that even the tiniest bones had a distinctive shape that resembled at least a portion of their adult counterparts.

The skull is incredibly difficult to understand in its infant form, and even adult skulls are tough to deal with when they're fragmented. Almost everyone can recognize the familiar shape of a complete human skull, but together the cranium and the face contain over two dozen separate components. Big, relatively flat bones form the back, top, and sides of the skull, with smaller, more complex bones surrounding the eyes and face. In decomposed or skeletonized infants, these bones are thin, incompletely formed, and not connected at all, looking more like big, irregular restaurant-style corn chips than human bones. Again,

Dr. Bass insisted that we know skull fragments backward and forward. He knew, and we were soon to learn, that the skull is a favorite target of murderers.

I must admit, it took me a while to hit my stride in osteology class—the way an anthropologist looks at bones is simply so different from the way an orthopedic surgeon views them. I was used to seeing bones live and whole, within a huge organic structure of which they were only a small though vital part—not as isolated elements that might be found scattered in a field or piled in the corner of a basement.

But once we moved from whole-bone identification to the analysis of fragments, my competitive spirit came through. My friend and fellow student, Tyler O'Brien, would sneak into the osteology lab with me each night, and we spent hours quizzing each other on every fragment in the collection. First we learned by sight—"Half of a right patella." "Portion of a lumbar vertebra." Then we shut our eyes and set ourselves to learning by touch alone the unique characteristics of each bone.

That process had taken months—but it had served us well. Both of us, as well as most of the class, could now take the merest glance at a whole bone and tell you what it was and which side of the body it came from. We could pick up the smallest fragment and find the key to its identity. Solving these intricate three-dimensional puzzles became a new and thrilling game.

Soon we were ready for an even more fascinating task—applying this knowledge to forensic anthropology analyses. Now, though, it was no longer a game. We were being taught to practice on real cases—albeit cases that had been solved years before. But our subjects were real people who had died violent deaths. It was up to us to figure out who they were and what had happened to them.

The routine was always the same. Dr. Bass would bring a collection of bones into the classroom on Tuesday morning, along with any pertinent case information, and leave everything there for a week. A skull, mandible, two thigh bones, and a section of pelvis might be piled on top of a tray along with the preliminary notes taken on the day the bones were found—for example, "Human skeletal remains found in a ditch along Alcoa Highway on July 7, 1987. No clothing was recovered." Then we had to analyze the remains, explaining what they told us about the victim's age, race, sex, stature, and any other clues we could come up with.

There were only about fifteen students in our class, so we split into teams of three or four and took turns examining the bones during the week and in our Thursday class. By the following Tuesday, we were each expected to produce a report—just like the ones we might turn in to a police investigation—telling the investigators everything we'd gleaned from our anthropologic examination. In fact, the class was as much about preparing the report as it was about analyzing the remains—no forensic anthropologist will last very long if he or she can't document evidence and share information with investigators— and it was made crystal clear from the beginning that we were to choose our words carefully and back up our opinions with good, hard science.

I was used to writing reports, of course, but only in the style of the medical records I had worked with at the clinic, in which a typical entry might state confidently, "This is a forty-five-year-old White female, 5'6" tall weighing 145 pounds." Of course, you could describe a whole body—living or dead—in that kind of detail. When all you've got is a skeleton, you can never be that specific, though you can usually come up with a more basic biological profile. For example:

BIOLOGICAL PROFILE: Case # 02–17

SEX:	Female
ESTIMATED AGE:	40 to 50 (within a range of 35 to 55)
RACE:	White
ESTIMATED STATURE:	5'5" to 5'7" (within a range of 5'3½" to 5'8")
WEIGHT:	Undetermined
SCALP HAIR:	Unknown

Every biological profile, Dr. Bass told us, would ideally include the anthropologist's "Big Four": sex, age, race, and stature. If you're lucky, and you've got the evidence to go further, you can put in ancillary information such as weight and maybe hair color. Often, human remains *do* survive with enough intact hair to determine color, because hair is made up of dead cells, which don't decompose as soft tissues do. Even a single long, blond hair found stuck to the underside of a skull can help tremendously when you are trying to identify skeletal remains.

Sometimes the associated evidence—evidence found with a body or remains—can give you a clue. Clothing, for example, can help you determine a person's weight and size, though, of course, it too tends to decompose. In the end, though, the bones last longest—and they hold many secrets if you know what to look for.

. . . .

One of the most basic ways we identify each other is by sex, so when I'm looking at newly discovered bones, I often start by asking myself whether they belonged to a man or a woman. Under these circumstances, I hope I've got at least part of the skull or the pelvis, because these bones possess the best morphological features to reveal the differences between male and female. ("Morphology" means the logic of shapes, the characteristics of a structure that can be seen but are difficult to measure.) Males, for instance, usually have a line of bone that juts out to form the "brow ridge," a horizontal ridge between their forehead and the tops of their eye sockets. This ridge is smaller, or absent entirely, in females. Males also have distinctive areas—much bigger than women's—for their large muscles to attach behind each ear and in the back of the head, near the hairline.

But it's the pelvis that really tells you about someone's sex. The pelvis is made up of three separate bones. At the bottom of the spine sits the sacrum, a wide, thick bone, shaped like a slice of pie and full of holes.

On either side sits the "innominate" or "no-name" bones, two relatively flat, softly curved slabs, each with a socket for one of the hip joints and a notch that allows the sciatic nerve to pass from the spine down into the leg. In females this sciatic notch begins to spread widely as a girl matures, while the front and back of a girl's pelvis becomes wider to accommodate the possible birth of a child. In men, the sciatic notch is narrower, as is the entire pelvis.

Overall, male skeletons tend to be larger and more robust than those of females, but there are exceptions to every rule. We've all met plenty of robust females and small, gracile males.

If sex is tricky to determine, age is really tough. After all, there are only two sexes—but a skeleton might be any age from 0 to 100. I personally have enough trouble telling the age of a living person, even when I can look at indicators like posture, hair color, and wrinkles.

Because exact age is so hard to figure, a forensic report usually gives age as an estimated range—say, thirty to forty in an adult; twelve to fifteen in a teenager or "subadult." Subadults' ages are easier to estimate, since their bones and teeth mature at a pretty steady and well-documented rate for the first fifteen or sixteen years. Then their bones undergo changes that are a little less predictable as they enter their early twenties. The bones usually don't get any bigger after that, but they do continue to mature until the middle to late twenties.

Age-related changes continue until the day we die, showing up in our ribs, pelvis, and weight-bearing joints—knees, hips, ankles, and spine. The ends of our ribs are stressed every time we take a breath, while the bones of our pelvis grate together throughout our entire lives. The amount of movement is usually so minuscule that we don't even notice it—yet over time that movement is enough to wear down the underlying bone in ways that an anthropologist can use to read a person's age.

Likewise, although the joining, or articulating, bones in the ankles, knees, hips, and spine are covered with a generous cushion of cartilage, sooner or later the cartilage wears down, leaving a record of every day we've stood upright and all the thousands of miles we've walked. And as the cartilage wears down, like the rubber on a tire, the underlying bone begins to show changes: first some irregularities around the edge of the joint, then some roughening of the gliding surfaces. With extreme age-related changes, the whole joint can appear to bubble and boil with bony convolutions, and the weight-bearing surfaces might even collapse.

Age-related changes aren't limited to the legs or spine. The arms, hands, and shoulders are also susceptible to disease and can also show lifelong signs of wear and tear. And then there are the teeth: Are they rugged and unstained? Well worn? Missing, with subsequent absorption of bone?

You'd think estimating a person's stature, or height, would be easiest of all, and you'd be right—if you had a complete body or the right bones. If all you've got is, say, a rib, you're out of luck. Stature can best be calculated from the leg bones, though the arm bones come in a good close second. The length of any of these bones can be entered into a mathematical formula which can then be used to calculate the stature of an individual within a limited range.

Finally, we come to race, a subject that can quickly become touchy and politically charged. For forensic anthropologists, though, race is less of a political topic than a matter of procedure: What can we find out about a mass of bones or body parts that will help police figure out who the person was? In our society, people tend to identify themselves by race, and their friends, family, and coworkers usually know them that way, too. So Dr. Bass made sure we knew the latest thinking on how skeletal structure might vary, depending on a person's racial background.

The bones of a person's mid-face—eye sockets, cheeks, nose, and mouth—reveal our ethnic heritage. For example, Negroid heritage is displayed in a skull with a wide, flattened opening for the nose, wide-set eye sockets, and a forward projecting set of upper and lower jaws. Likewise, a long, narrow nose with a high-pitched nasal bridge and oval-shaped eye orbits tells me that the skull probably belonged to a Caucasian, while in someone of Asian parentage, I would expect to see relatively flat cheekbones and a nose whose characteristics fall some-where between Negroids and Caucasians—neither flat nor high-bridged.

To learn all of this had taken us months—but by the time Dr. Bass threw his latest challenge at us, we'd all gotten pretty good and he knew it. Yet as he'd given us this week's collection of bones, his words had had the ring of triumph: "In twenty years, no one has ever gotten this one right." Why not? It seemed to me that every one of us could have measured the bones on the tray, identified the morphological traits, and then told him that we were looking at a tall, well-muscled White man in his sixties. Why would such a simple problem have stumped students for the past two decades?

It was Friday night before I found my way back to the lab where Tyler and I worked together, measuring each bone and documenting our findings. We'd learned through the grapevine that our conclusions didn't differ from anyone else's. Yet I just couldn't shake the feeling that I was missing something.

The night before my report was due, I returned yet again to the lab. I ran my fingers over the contours of the bones and stared at them for hours in the semi-trancelike stillness that was often where I got my best ideas.

And then, suddenly, I *knew.* I couldn't say how. But I finally under-stood the secret answer hidden within this apparently simple problem. I hurried home and spent the rest of the night writing my report.

·   ·   ·

The next day, Dr. Bass collected our reports and began his usual oral questioning. "How many think this skeleton was male?"

Every hand in the room went up.

"Middle-aged?"

Unanimous again.

"About six feet tall, plus or minus an inch or two?"

Yes again.

"White?"

Every hand in the room rose—except mine.

"Miss Craig?" said Dr. Bass. He was always so courteous and formal, I couldn't tell whether he was surprised or not.

"I think the man was Black," I said into the sudden silence.

Could it be that Dr. Bass was actually at a loss for words? For a moment, he just stared at me. Then he laughed, the way he usually did when one of us got it wrong, and my heart sank. Finally, he sighed.

"Well," he said, drawing out his words for emphasis. "I never thought I'd see the day." He shook his head and picked up a photo from his desk—a picture of the person whose bones these were. He was indeed male, middle-aged, tall—and Black. My classmates looked at each other and then at me.

Dr. Bass interrogated me further when we met in his office. "Miss Craig," he asked me, "how did you know the man was Black?"

I tried to recall exactly what I had seen last night in the lab, which specific detail had triggered my flash of insight.

"It was his knees," I said finally. "The joint just *looks* Black."

Dr. Bass ran his hand across his buzz-cut, looking for all the world like the frazzled D.A. on *Perry Mason.* "You may somehow have stumbled upon the right answer, Miss Craig," he said sternly. "But your work will never stand up in court if you can't prove what you know."

.   .   .

All right. How could I prove what I knew? Lucky for me, I found this an interesting problem, because it was a challenge that would recur again and again throughout my career: I'd have a flash of insight that would seem to descend mysteriously from nowhere, something I'd just *know* was true without being able to say how. Then I'd have to do the hard scientific labor of reconstructing the unconscious processes that had produced the insight, working backward from solution to proof. I don't think my instinct has ever steered me wrong—but sometimes finding the proof can be difficult.

The general scientific basis for my discovery, of course, was something we'd all learned together in class. Once Dr. Bass had taught us the rules for determining race from bone, he'd gone on to explain that skeletal evidence doesn't always correlate with the color of a person's skin, or the texture of their hair, or even the continent they call home. The Caucasian bones in any given face might belong to a person of coffee-colored skin who identifies as Cuban or Latino or even African American. The owner of a skull with Negroid characteristics might have pale creamy skin and come from a family that considers itself Puerto Rican. Bones tell some of the story—but not all of it.

In this case, though, all I'd had to look at was the bones—and somehow I'd gotten it right. So what had tipped me off? The first clue I'd had to this man's race was when I'd looked at his femur, or thigh bone. Earlier that year, I'd learned that among Caucasoids—the scientific term for Whites—the femur demonstrates a forward bowing of the shaft, known to anthropologists as "anterior [forward] curvature." In Black people—Negroids—the femur is relatively straight. The femur in Dr. Bass's assignment had been curved—and yet I had known the man was Black. How?

I decided to take a closer look at some femurs. Off I went to Bass's collection of bones, where I lined up twenty male right femurs—ten White males, ten Black—spacing them apart like railroad ties on the shiny black lab table. Slowly an idea began to grow. Maybe it wasn't the femur's shaft I'd been responding to, but the bone's distal end, the end that fits into the knee.

Was this one of those times when I had to rely on touch as well as sight? Closing my eyes, I ran my fingers slowly down to the notch at the distal end. First the White femurs. Then the Black ones . . .

Wait a minute—here was something! I opened my eyes. Now I could see it. The difference was in the intercondylar notch, the place at the center of the knee joint where the thigh fits into the knee. There was a marked racial difference in the angle of the notch—and somehow, without even realizing it, that was what I'd noticed.

By the time I was ready to graduate in the summer of 1994, I was able to prove that, on the average, the angle of the intercondylar notch differs by about 10 degrees between Blacks and Whites. And I'd come to understand why a generation of Dr. Bass's students had failed at the case I'd finally solved. Because of racial mixing in this country, many African Americans (and probably lots of Whites, too) have a variety of racial characteristics. Our test case's White heritage could be read in the bones of his skull and the curve of his thigh bones—clues to which we had all responded. But the angle of his intercondylar notch revealed his Black ancestry as well.

I was coming to see for myself that skin color doesn't necessarily line up with bone evidence. Our test case might have been light-skinned, dark-skinned, or anything in between, with bones that said one thing and hair and skin that hinted at another. This wasn't the last time I was almost fooled. In 1997, for instance, when I was working as the Commonwealth of Kentucky's forensic anthropologist, I helped to recover a decomposed body from a cistern in Campbell County. Visually, it seemed that these remains had once belonged to a female with straight, reddish-brown hair and skin the color of dirty snow, so we gave local newspapers and TV stations a description of this missing White female, hoping that someone who knew her would come forward.

After weeks of no response, I agreed to do a three-dimensional facial reconstruction on this woman's skull—and as soon as I removed all of the flesh and saw her facial bones, I realized that our ID had gone awry. This woman's skull demonstrated evidence of racial admixture—that combination of White and Black parentage that leaves nature a lot of choices as to skin color, hair texture, and facial features. When we changed our description to "mixed race," we were finally able to find someone who knew this person—a dark-skinned woman whose friends considered her "mixed race." It seemed the six months she spent in the cistern had been enough to destroy her dark epidermal (outer) layer of skin, leaving only the pigment-free endodermal (inner) layer, a creamy white covering dotted with gray patches from the decomposition. Without the skeletal evidence, we would never have found out who she was.

· · ·

Once we students had some training under our belts, we were sent out into the field as part of a forensic team that worked on actual Tennessee cases under Dr. Bass's supervision. This arrangement had been carefully worked out between the school and law enforcement agencies throughout the state, and it was an invaluable part of our training. Just as in class, all of our case findings had to be written in a concise report that could be read and understood by the wide range of local, state, and federal investigators who might be interested. We also knew that we might have to testify in court, explaining what we'd found in language that a jury could follow and defending our opinions against a defense attorney's challenges.

No longer were we doing this work for academic credit alone. Now it was for real, and the demands on us were high. We couldn't just state that a young woman had sustained a high-velocity gunshot wound to the side of her head—we had to describe the gross and microscopic appearance of the wound: How had her skull bone been damaged? At what point had the bullet entered? What did the hole look like? How did we know it was an entrance wound (where the bullet went in) and not an exit wound (where the bullet went out)? Then we had to back up our findings by citing documented studies of similar wounds.

Despite the simplified, positive statements that fictional detectives tend to make, we learned to pepper our reports with such cautious phrases as "most likely," "consistent with," and "appears to be." And we made sure to back up every opinion we offered with citations from peer-reviewed scientific articles. Slowly but surely, we learned to avoid speculation about the actual murder scenario, limiting ourselves to strictly clinical terms and standard anatomical nomenclature. Let the TV scientists proclaim that *"The victim was crouched on the floor when the killer grabbed her hair and then shot her with a gun held six inches from her left ear—making him, of course, right-handed."* In the real world, such a report would more likely read: *"There is a circular defect one inch anterior to the left external auditory meatus. This defect is eleven millimeters in diam-*

eter and demonstrates internal beveling. Internal beveling is characteristic of entrance gunshot wounds to the skull. [Here we would insert a citation referring to the appropriate portion of the scientific literature.] *There is no evidence of gunpowder stippling in the bone."*

Although we were learning volumes from this on-the-job training, our professors warned us not to cut classes to work on a case. But by now we only had four or five hours of formal lectures each week, so we were usually able to respond quickly whenever we were called to a crime scene. Our team was loosely organized, drawn from a pool of about ten grad students, with a core group of half a dozen willing to be on call 24–7 to every law enforcement agency in the state of Tennessee.

Dr. Bass often went with us. But even when he wasn't physically present, we knew that the responsibility was ultimately his. As lead investigator, he would review everything we did and his signature would be above ours in every report. If we screwed up, you could bet we'd hear about it—but if we did well, we'd hear about that, too, and that was what kept us going. Once again, I had cause to be grateful for Dr. Bass's demanding standards, because it was this experience that really taught me how to think like a detective, how to use my common sense, instinct, and intuition as well as my book-learning.

Almost every case started with a visit to the crime scene. We never heard about the "fresh" bodies—that was a job for the pathologist. But if they found decomposing remains, unassociated body parts, or bones, they'd call in the anthropologists.

We'd rush to the scene—perhaps a farmhouse with two smoking corpses or maybe a back-alley apartment with a cache of bones hidden under the floorboards. We'd check in with the officer in charge, who would already have secured the scene. Then we'd work with the officers to come up with a plan for gathering and documenting the evidence.

Here is where I learned how crucial is the information gleaned from the scene. Sure, lab analysis was vitally important, but every investigation starts with the crime scene—if only you know how to look.

On one very early case, I, the novice, saw nothing out of the ordinary until fellow student Bill Grant pointed out that the charred body
in the car was covered with burned maggots. This was irrefutable evidence that the man, and his car, had been torched well *after* he had
started to decompose.

In another case, the sheriff took me aside and told me that our murder suspect had just confessed to beating the victim to death with a golf
club. I realized how close I might have come to disregarding the broken putter we'd just found in our search through a roadside dump for
scattered bones.

Yet another time, I was initially led astray when I examined a
severely decomposed and partially skeletonized body propped up
against a tree with her legs splayed in a provocative pose—a location
that could be easily seen from a nearby road. I assumed that the victim
had died there—until I found another site, about fifteen feet away, that
contained her teeth, a portion of her broken jaw, pieces of her jewelry,
and a mat of her scalp hair, which had sloughed off during the early
stages of decomposition. Clearly, someone had moved the dead girl and
propped her up in a perverse attempt to display her to passersby. I figured this one out after about two hours of careful analysis, but next
time I'd know not to make any quick assumptions about where and
how someone had died until I had thoroughly investigated the entire
crime scene.

Once we'd learned everything we could from the scene, we'd take
the evidence back with us to the university lab, covering every piece
of evidence with the paper trail known in law enforcement circles as
the "chain of custody." Whenever any piece of evidence changed
hands, someone had to sign and date a piece of paper indicating who
was taking it and where it was going.

Back at the lab, we'd begin the second phase of the analysis. Our job
was most often to help the police identify victims, offering basic information that would enable police to request someone's medical records
or talk to a family in search of a positive ID. Police also asked us to help
determine time of death—pathologists could do that from intact soft

tissue remaining on whole fresh corpses, but we anthropologists were becoming specialists in analyzing decaying flesh, charred tissue, and bone.

We were fortunate to have the decay facility as a reference resource. For example, say we had a case where skeletal remains were found still encased in a flannel shirt and denim jeans. We could turn to documentation from studies of corpses dressed in similar garments, learning how long it had taken for the clothes to rot away to the point where they matched the victim's. If we had a decomposing body, we could turn to Bass's notes on research projects documenting the rate and pattern of postmortem tooth loss; of maggot infestation; and of soft-tissue decomposition, liquefaction, and eventual disappearance.

Every day we were finding answers to new questions, and each answer led to still more questions: How long does it take for the plants surrounding a corpse to discolor, die, and then return with vigor? Do the bloodier corpses affect plants differently than the ones that are relatively intact? How long does it take for a person's hair to fall out—and under what kind of circumstances will it fall out faster? What if an animal uses this hair in its nest—how far away should you look for that and how do you recognize it? Does the hair change color after death? What if it's gotten contaminated with rotting flesh and animal feces—how can you tell and what should you look for? We learned to ask these and a thousand other questions—and, slowly but surely, we learned to answer them, answers that I put to good use working the rest of the cases in this book.

.　.　.

What brought it all together for me was what I like to think of as the "Friends and Family Case of 1993." It all began when the Grainger County rescue squad pulled Richard Carpenter's relatively fresh body out of a cistern. No, amend that: They pulled out *most* of his body, but his head and his penis were missing. Tennessee State Medical Examiner Dr. Cleland Blake called our team from the backyard of a farmhouse in Bean Station, up in the northeast corner of Tennessee. The victim's head and penis were probably still in the cistern, he told us. But no one could say for sure.

The detectives were already putting a case together against Donald Ferguson, whose arrest warrant alleged that he had "slipped up behind" his longtime friend Richard and "hit him in the head with a hammer." Donald then reportedly cut off Richard's head and penis with the electric carving knife that hung by the kitchen door in the tiny frame house that Donald shared with his mother. As reported in the *Knoxville News-Sentinel,* Donald's mother, Nannie, had heard a "thump" in the night. The next day she saw Richard's body in the backyard and his head in a plastic bag.

Nannie, who had suffered repeated psychological and physical abuse from her son, was severely beaten by him once more. Instead of cowering in submission as she had done so many times, she fled directly to the Grainger County Sheriff's Department and filed a complaint. "I've got bruises all over my body . . . and I've been wanting to talk about this," she said. She also told authorities that Donald had put the body in the cistern.

County D.A. Al Schmutzer thought the murder had occurred on Thursday night, August 19. On Friday morning, when Grainger County deputies arrived at his house, Donald was, as always, out front with a broom, tidying things up. Richard Carpenter's truck was still in the driveway and his mixed-breed dog was still standing guard over it. The bewildered dog wandered off that afternoon, never to be seen again.

Later that day, volunteer members of the local fire and rescue squad pulled the body from the cistern, and Dr. Blake called us. He'd seen the cut marks on the victim's neck bones, and he expected to find matching cut marks on the vertebrae still attached to the head. He wanted anthropologists to document that these marks did indeed match and then to help him further match the cut marks to a specific knife or saw.

Just as my classmates Tom Bodkin, Lee Meadows-Jantz, and I pulled up in our big white truck, volunteers were lifting the plastic bag containing the victim's head out of the water with a grappling hook, while the deputies watched from the farmhouse's back door, smoking cigarettes and drinking coffee. We joined them, expecting to be steered toward the newly discovered head. But after we all exchanged the pleasantries that are a cultural requirement in the South, the deputies escorted us into the suspect's bedroom.

When they arrested Ferguson, they told us, they'd insisted that he empty his pockets and spread the contents on his bed. There among his keys and loose change was a human kneecap. This patella appeared to have acquired a smooth polish, the kind it might have gotten from the skin oils and regular rubbing of a human hand. And indeed, Ferguson told the deputies, he'd been carrying the patella in his pocket for the past year. Then he told us even more—he'd thrown his wife, Shirley, into the cistern after beating her to death two years earlier. He'd made up a story about her running off with another man and, until now, everyone had believed him.

By now Ferguson was at the local jail and was no longer cooperating with the authorities. So Tom, Lee, and I gathered in the yard with Dr. Blake, the men from the Tennessee Bureau of Investigation (TBI), the sheriff's department, and the local rescue workers.

"We already searched the yard and outbuildings when we were looking for Richard," one burly deputy explained. He added that he and his colleagues had found tiny bits of blood spattered on the kitchen walls and floor despite the obvious lengths to which someone had gone to clean up the crime scene. So, he went on, investigators had kept searching until they found the patella in Ferguson's pocket. Now, despite his confession, they needed us to confirm that the object was indeed a human bone. Yes, Lee told him. It was. Clearly there were more skeletal remains to be found, so we formed teams to look for them—one for the house, a second for the yard and outbuildings, and a third to drain the cistern.

Cisterns are an integral part of homes throughout Appalachia. The rural areas don't always have sewers or water services, and it's usually too expensive to sink a well. If someone living in the country wants water, he or she pretty much has to collect rainwater or bring in a truckload of water to fill the cistern—a large, concrete-lined hole or a polyvinylchloride (PVC) drum buried in the ground, about three feet wide at the top, six to eight feet wide at the bottom, and up to twelve feet deep.

Detectives hadn't yet had to enter Ferguson's concrete cistern— they'd used ropes and grappling hooks to retrieve Carpenter's body and then his head. But if there were more bones down there, a grappling hook wouldn't be enough. As we made our plans, Dr. Blake let us see the head, which he'd already photographed. There, in the victim's mouth, was the bloody stump of an amputated penis. As we stood staring at it, the rescue workers continued to drag the cistern with a net, retrieving a few plastic bags, a rotting shirt, and a single bone, which one of the firefighters held high over his head and waved in the air. All of us anthropologists could see right away that it was a radius—a bone from the human forearm.

"Okay," I heard myself saying. "Now we know Ferguson was telling the truth. We'll have to drain the cistern." Much to my surprise, the words came out with a tone of authority that sounded confident even to me. I expected the other investigators to cock their heads and smirk at the "uppity new kid," but they only nodded in agreement and asked my advice on how to retrieve the rest of the bones without damaging any critical evidence.

Suddenly, everyone was looking at me. Lee was actually the most experienced member of the team, with Tom still a newcomer. But by age, I appeared to be the senior member of our team, so folks seemed to assume that I'd be the one to come up with something.

I knew that someday I'd be out of school, and then I really would be in charge of recovery efforts like this one. I felt so ill-equipped— and I knew that the investigative team in Ferguson's yard had decades of training and experience. Surely the local firefighters knew more about cisterns than I did. And clearly the detectives had amassed years of experience searching for and documenting evidence.

So I came up with an approach that I still rely on today: I gathered the leaders of each team and drew on their strengths. "All right, gentlemen," I said to the sheriff's chief deputy, the lead man from TBI, the volunteer fire chief, and Dr. Blake, the M.E. "Let's work together to set up a plan. We need to get all the water out of that cistern, but we can't disturb or lose any evidence. What do *you* think is the best way to get it done?"

To my delight, this method worked. The team members immediately began offering suggestions—for my approval. For the first time I could remember, my relatively advanced age was working for me—at the ripe old age of forty-five, I at least *looked* like someone who should be in charge. Some of the TBI detectives had worked with me before and they knew I was still a student. But they also knew that I'd been working with Dr. Bass for almost three years, serving as a key investigator in some of his recent major cases. They were clearly willing to trust my judgment, making me think that I should trust it, too.

I started with the team that was going to drain the cistern. The local fire department had figured out how to pump the water out, so I made only one small suggestion: Put a screen over the outflow pipe to catch any small particles or bones that might be sucked out with the water. They improvised, pulling a screen from an outbuilding's window and propping it up on concrete blocks. A few minutes later, we found our first prize: some small human hand bones.

Lee was now busy over at a dump site at the property's edge, where she'd found what looked like another piece of bone in a pile of ashes. She'd found a chunk of parietal bone from the side of a skull—and to everyone's bewilderment, there seemed to be a neat round hole right in the middle of it. Detailed analysis of *that* would have to wait, however, as Lee and I were suddenly being summoned to examine the contents of the wood-burning stove in the living room. Sure enough, there were bones inside the stove, which we'd now have to dismantle and search.

Not yet, however, because just then, another detective who had been searching the kitchen called out to me. He had found still more bones—in the kitchen cupboard, propped up on a plastic canister beside a glass that held a toothbrush and a tube of toothpaste. At first he'd thought the items were soup bones, or maybe bones set aside for some dog—but I saw at a glance that he'd found two human heel bones and a piece of a breastbone, or sternum. Like the bone in the trash pile, the sternum had a neat round hole right through the middle. What in the hell was going on here?

No sooner had I identified these bones as being human than another firefighter came rushing in from draining the cistern.

"The water is almost all out, and you won't believe what we've got down there, Doc," he cried out. "It looks like almost a whole skeleton!"

The discovery didn't surprise me—but being called "Doc" did. I'm sure it happened just because the volunteer didn't know my name. But even though I didn't yet have a right to the title, I didn't correct him. After all, I didn't want to embarrass him, did I?

From that point on, things kept happening faster and faster. When I looked down into the cistern, I saw dozens of human bones, all jumbled up on the bottom. If they had seemed to mirror the victim's position at death—stretched out prone, huddled against a wall, or bound hand and foot—we would have had to document their position. Since they were so clearly in disarray, though, we decided simply to send someone down into the cistern to retrieve them. (Later I wondered what the murderer and his mother did about their drinking water. Maybe they thought the bones gave it an interesting flavor. At any rate, the decomposing body didn't seem to have affected their health—or not so they noticed.)

Of course, getting into the cistern was harder than it sounded. Whoever went down there would be working in a confined underground space where a body had been rotting, producing gases and other toxins. The fire chief insisted that anyone who entered the cistern had to wear a self-contained breathing apparatus (SCBA) tank and respirator, adding to the sense of danger. Finally, Tom agreed to take on the job.

Meanwhile, Lee and I had other work to do. Searchers were finding bones all over the property, and we were being called over to inspect their findings in the yard, behind the barn, in and under the outbuildings. Luckily all of these new discoveries turned out to be animal bones—some from table scraps fed to the dogs, some from rabbits, rats, opossums, and cats that had apparently died some time ago. However, there were still plenty of human bones in the cistern, the stove, and the cupboard.

Eventually, it grew dark, so we secured the scene for the night, stringing crime scene tape around the property and putting a sheriff's deputy on guard to keep civilians out. But the next morning, as we pulled onto the small road that led up to the Ferguson farm, we found it jammed with the cars and pickup trucks of local residents. Word about the murders had traveled quickly and our crime scene had turned into a Saturday-morning picnic, with residents setting up their lawn chairs, opening up their picnic baskets, and playing with their children.

"I don't believe it," I said under my breath to Lee. But she had grown up in this area and she just shook her head.

"Around here, that's par for the course," she drawled. "Can't say as I blame them. It's cheaper than a movie."

So for the rest of the day, we had an audience. They called out encouragement to us when we started sifting an area that Ferguson had used as a dump, and they let out a loud cheer when detectives dismantled the wood-burning stove and brought it out into the yard so that Lee and I could sift the ashes. Lee was about seven months pregnant at the time, and as she bent over the sifting screen, one of the onlookers called out an offer of his folding lawn chair.

"Why not?" Lee called back. "Thanks!" When I offered to walk over and get the chair, a little girl came running over with a chair for me, too. Lee and I went back to work, sifting ashes in relative comfort while the crowd ate their picnic lunches and country music blared from the radio on a nearby pickup.

Later that day, deputies brought Ferguson to the scene and began questioning him about where he'd put the rest of his wife's remains. So far, we'd found her bones mixed in with his pocket change, in the cistern, in the kitchen cupboard, in the stove, and in a trash dump. But some bones were still missing, and the deputy suggested that I question him myself.

I had never knowingly spoken to a murder suspect before, but I was willing to give it a try. I don't know what I expected, but in a million years, I'd never have guessed what Ferguson said when I asked him where the bones were.

"Oh," he said calmly, "I pulled them out of the cistern and burned them for fuel this winter. It got pretty cold out here." Amazingly, he knew the name of every bone and gave me a detailed description of which ones he'd hidden in the kitchen, as opposed to those he'd put in his bedroom. Not only that, but he cleared up the mystery of the holes. In apparent fits of loneliness, he would retrieve one of his wife's bones from the cistern and drill a hole in it just big enough to thread with a long leather thong. Then he'd wear it around his neck, giving a whole new meaning to the term "trophy wife."

Ferguson also assured us that we had scoured all of his hiding places (and he eventually pled guilty to both murders). We had enough evidence to convict him and enough bones to identify the victim, so detectives from the TBI told us to go home.

As Lee and I packed up our gear and made our way back to our truck, the crowd of onlookers started to applaud. To them, we weren't just dirty, tired forensic anthropology students. We were some kind of heroes.

Lee and I looked at each other and laughed. At this point I wasn't worried about an inappropriate reaction. What *would* be an appropriate reaction in a situation like this?

But I'd turned over an important page in my professional development there in Bean Station, Tennessee. For the first time, I'd been considered the lead investigator on the forensic anthropology team. Experienced investigators had turned to me for direction and I was forced to make quick decisions that—right or wrong—would affect the investigation's outcome. I felt that I had passed a final, crucial test— a test that I now realized I'd be taking over and over and over again. There would never be a rule book at any crime scene I processed. I'd have to rely on common sense, academic training, and the ability to improvise—just as I had done here.

But next time I'd bring my own lawn chair.

3

Waco

The evil that men do lives after them;
the good is oft interred with their bones.
— WILLIAM SHAKESPEARE

T
HERE ARE *two torsos in this bag!"*
"I have a baby's hand—who needs a baby's hand?"
"Does that foot match my leg?"

We were calling out in the morgue, but we could barely hear over the whining bone saws, clanking metal trays, and roaring industrial-strength garbage disposals. The smell of burned bone and tissue flooded my nostrils until I thought I could taste it, but I tried to stay as focused as all the other professionals here, the blood-spattered pathologists, anthropologists, and dentists busily sorting through the scraps and shards—the remains of the people who had once called themselves the Branch Davidians.

Two months before, they had been a community of men, women, and children living in relative secrecy in Mount Carmel, their guarded enclave on the outskirts of Waco, Texas. Today, they were body parts in the morgue. Their fate was the end result of a series of miscalculations and violent acts that will never be completely justified or understood. Now, though, I was part of a team seeking to discover who they were and how they had died. At least we could do that.

· · · ·

It all started with Vernon Howell, better known as David Koresh, who led a cult that he named for himself—the Branch Davidians. The charismatic Koresh had ruled his community with an iron hand, prescribing harsh punishments for wayward souls. He persuaded the Davidians to move into the Waco compound, isolating themselves from the sinful world. He also persuaded them to give him everything they owned, using their wealth to amass a huge cache of illegal weapons—his defense against what he saw as the Bible's promise of imminent apocalypse.

It was this mass of firearms and explosives that drew the attention of the Bureau of Alcohol, Tobacco and Firearms (ATF), which duly sent agents to the compound with a search warrant. But as the ATF agents moved in, the Davidians opened fire from the compound's windows, doors, and rooftops, killing four agents and wounding more than a dozen. As the ATF returned fire, five Davidians were also killed, and Koresh himself was wounded.

The Davidians barricaded themselves inside the compound and a fifty-one-day siege began. The Federal Bureau of Investigation (FBI) replaced the ATF as the lead agency and tried to convince the Davidians to surrender themselves peacefully. A few did leave the compound—but most stayed locked inside.

Finally, the FBI turned to desperate measures. On the morning of April 19, 1993, they used tanks to punch holes in the compound walls and pumped in clouds of tear gas, hoping to flush the Davidians out into the open. Instead, the Davidians stood their ground and began to shoot until the FBI backed off. Then they doused their own compound with fuel and set it on fire. Within minutes, wind-whipped flames were roaring through the ramshackle buildings, igniting the stockpiles of ammunition. The resulting explosions created huge mushroom-shaped clouds of fire and smoke worthy of the holocaust that Koresh predicted. When the smoke cleared, some eighty people were dead.

•   •   •

I watched the fire mesmerized on the small television I kept in my office, its tiny screen filled with flames. The news reporters tried desperately to keep up with the contradictory reports: No Davidians were coming out of the building—was that because they wouldn't or because they couldn't? What about reports of gunshots coming from inside the compound as it burned? Were the Davidians firing wildly at the FBI—or was it simply the heat of the fire, exploding the ammunition allegedly stored there on-site?

One thing was obvious: No one could survive that inferno. My fellow anthropology students and I watched for hours as the number of presumed victims rose to sixty, seventy, eighty . . .

When mass disasters strike today, authorities call in an elite squad of trained death investigators under the auspices of such organizations as DMORT (Disaster Mortuary Operational Response Team). But in 1993, there was no national structure, and the morgue work fell to local medical examiners, who had to call on their own personal network of experts if they needed extra help. Since our own Dr. Bill Bass was world-famous for his skill in victim identification, we knew he'd be asked to help out at Waco. Every forensic anthropology grad student in the department hoped to be taken with him.

After years of working fire-related death scenes as part of Bass's team, we could all picture what was involved. The bodies of the Davidians had undoubtedly burned beyond the point of recognition, or even customary identification procedures such as fingerprints. To identify their remains—to put names on their graves—someone would have to gather the bone shards and teeth and skull fragments scattered amid the rubble, hoping to find enough bits and pieces to match previously existing medical and dental records.

Even small, quickly extinguished structure fires can kill, causing a victim to die of smoke inhalation with little visible injury. A little more time in the fire makes the skin blister and the eyes and tongue swell. The victims might be dead and slightly disfigured, but you can still tell who they are. Usually, though, a fire is far more brutal.

The scalp is the first to go, as the hair quickly turns to ashes. In a matter of seconds, the facial skin blisters, then splits, shrinks, and burns to a crisp. That thin layer by which we recognize each other is quickly consumed by flames that leave only a hard blackened mask across the cheeks and jaw. And forget about tattoos, scars, or birthmarks—anything that might be used to identify a victim—because they disappear without a trace.

Next, the muscles start to burn. Then the bones. Body parts with little or no soft tissue coverings burn first: head, fingers, toes, hands, feet. Minutes after the head becomes a skull, the arms and legs turn into dry, almost mummified cylinders of muscle and bone.

The lower spine, thighs, and pelvis are more durable. Solid, heavy bones covered with relatively large masses of soft tissue, they can last longer than any other part of the body. Meanwhile, the fire's warmth envelops the stomach and chest, causing the organs and intestines to expand even as the skin starts to shrink and split. As a result, the internal organs will sometimes burst through the abdomen, erupting out of the belly like some sci-fi alien, the blood curdling and boiling as it, too, escapes the walls of its vessels.

After an hour or so, only bones are left. But not those pristine white skeletons that you may have seen hanging in the corner of an anatomy lab. Bone in its natural state is a pale, buttery yellow. Toasted in the heat of a raging fire, it turns brown, then black, blue-gray, gray, white and, finally, ash. The smaller bones go through those stages quickly, though if you're lucky you might come upon the ashes in an almost cartoon-like state, holding the bone's original size and shape until the slightest gust of wind or careless touch sends them crumbling into dust.

Even the sturdiest bones tend to warp and fracture after the insulating muscles and skin are burned off. The skull goes especially quickly once the thin protective covering of the scalp has burned away, so that the bone is directly exposed to the heat. The skull tends to split as the brain inside heats up, building up a head of steam that eventually bursts through the fragile burned bones. But even the skull that survives the cooking of the brain is likely to shatter after prolonged exposure to the heat.

By the time the fire has done its work, those bones that have not yet been reduced to ash may have lost all connection to organic matter, so that only their mineral salts remain. (Those salts—from animal bones—are what give bone china its strong yet delicate texture.) The technical term for this reduction to brittle white mineral is "calcination." In a very short time, a 180-pound human body can be burnt down to a few pounds of calcined bone and some scraps of blackened muscle.

But let's not forget the teeth, made from the body's strongest tissue. False teeth, of course, are long gone by this time, but well after the hips and spine have been reduced to ashy fragments, a person's natural teeth may remain—to the undying gratitude of forensic investigators. Of course, burnt teeth become brittle and the enamel is likely to separate from the root. And if the surrounding bone has burned away, as often happens, the tooth fragments tend to fall down into the debris. Still, if you sift diligently and long enough, you are likely to find at least one or two dental clues in even the most vicious fire.

In fact, teeth usually survive even a professional crematory, along with some fragments of the larger bones. That's why professional cremationists don't trust entirely to fire—they take the burnt remains and put them in a pulverizer, which grinds the bone shards and broken teeth into ash and fragments small enough to fit in an urn. Luckily for forensic investigators, any fire—even an inferno as devastating as the one at Waco—will leave bone fragments and teeth.

I could well imagine the arduous recovery process that had begun at

Waco as soon as the smoke had cleared, with forensic investigators of all types kneeling in the rubble, sifting through the ashes and debris. What a horrifying job! Not only would these victims be burned truly beyond recognition, but their remains would be all mixed together—"commingled," as we call it. I pictured the families in those ramshackle, crowded buildings, pressed together in a wild dash for the exit, trying to escape the flames, or maybe huddled in places they thought would provide safety. And when the fire had reduced their bodies to fragile clumps of burned bone and muscle, parts from one person would almost certainly have broken off to mix with the burned parts of another—an arm thrown over a leg, a torso tumbling down to lie beside a skull. Pieces of the buildings would have crashed down upon the burning corpses, breaking off more body parts, as the intense heat of the fire melted skin onto muscle and fused tissue onto charred bone. Burned wood, nails, and debris would have joined the mix of flesh and ashes to form a homogenous black mass of charcoal, punctuated only by splintery bones and scattered teeth.

So investigators would do their best to extract the human remains from this mass of debris, sorting it as best they could on the spot and then shipping it over to the local morgue, which happened to be the Tarrant County facility in Fort Worth. (Even though the Waco catastrophe had taken place in McClennan County, the medical examiner's office in neighboring Tarrant County was under contract to do McClennan's autopsies.) Usually, a morgue is staffed only with pathologists—experts who analyze soft tissue and perform autopsies on a regular basis. But the soft tissue of most of these eighty or more people had been reduced to ash and charcoal. Time to call in the forensic dentists and anthropologists to look at the teeth and bone.

Had this been a "normal" multi-fatality fire—say, an out-of-control grease fire in a crowded bar or social club—investigators would already be facing a challenging and intricate death investigation as they sought to assemble each set of remains and give it a name. But this was no ordinary fire—it had been set, deliberately, in the midst of a controversial law enforcement effort that had drawn an enormous amount of media coverage. So the team at Fort Worth would also be conducting a very visible criminal investigation, treating each scrap of bone and shred of tissue as pieces of evidence. The anthropologists permitted at the scene would need to know more than academic science—they'd also have to know how to observe confidentiality mandates and chain-of-custody protocols. In Knoxville, we spelled that mixture of anthropological and forensic expertise "B-A-S-S."

But Dr. Bass's wife had just died of cancer, and he was in the throes of settling her affairs. Reluctantly, he decided to stay in Knoxville, sending graduate students to go in his place. To our mingled pride, excitement, and apprehension, he chose Bill Grant, Theresa Woltanski—and me.

●   ●   ●

The three of us piled into my vintage Jeep Cherokee, throwing an odd assortment of clothes, food, and field gear into the back. If we were assigned to the morgue—analyzing the remains as they came in—we'd be issued the normal protective gear: scrubs, gloves, and masks. But if we were assigned to recover remains at the site itself, we'd need to supply our own clothes: work boots, hats, foul-weather gear, and specialized excavation tools. We were taking no chances on showing up unprepared.

We drove all night and showed up in Fort Worth at six a.m.—just one hour before we'd been asked to meet Chief Medical Examiner Dr. Nazim Peerwani in his office. We knew from experience that we wouldn't be allowed to just walk in. A medical examiner's office is almost always secreted behind locked doors and security checkpoints, with carefully controlled access to the public. After all, behind those locked doors, the M.E.'s staff is trying to piece together the stories of the most personal and violent crimes. Distraught families, often ready to lash out at any target, tend to show up at the M.E.'s office, and sometimes perpetrators show up there too, perhaps driven by some irrational urge to further punish their dead victims, hoping to destroy key evidence of their crime, or even seeking to preserve their freedom by killing or disabling one of the scientific sleuths working on their case.

In a mass-fatality incident, with dozens of family members showing up to identify the dead, it's even more important to control access to the morgue. Medical examiners, hoping to shield families from the horrors of a charred body or disfigured face, want very much to control civilians' access to the remains, even as family members insist on seeing their loved ones one last time. Influenced by TV images, many civilians imagine a morgue as a kind of clinical funeral home, with neat rows of peacefully sleeping corpses—as opposed to the blood-spattered and often chaotic place of business that it is.

It's also important to keep out the thrill-seekers who inevitably congregate at disaster sites, their morbid curiosity fueled by the media and occasionally evolving into a fanatical desire to penetrate behind closed doors. Ordinarily rational, well-mannered people suddenly start behaving like spectators at a Roman circus, insisting on their very own up-close-and-personal view of the dead bodies as they appear on TV.

So although Bill, Theresa, and I had not yet worked a mass fatality, we weren't surprised when the large, polite man from the county sheriff's department stopped us as soon as we stepped off the sidewalk.

"Dr. Peerwani is expecting us! Please let us through!" Theresa said impatiently. One of my closest friends in the program, she was always quick to confront any perceived injustice. Now her long blond hair whipped across her sleep-deprived face as she spoke urgently to the officer.

"At least call Dr. Peerwani on your radio," Bill suggested. A tall, easygoing military veteran who seldom got worked up over anything, he was my other close buddy and, as it happened, Theresa's boyfriend. I looked at him gratefully, glad for his diplomatic skills and his air of quiet authority.

Eventually, we were taken to a reception area where we were issued special identification badges printed right then and there—good for this incident only. Anyone who wanted access to the morgue had to wear one of these highly visible badges at all times.

"Hold on there, folks," the receptionist said as we headed for the next locked door. "Y'all will have to wait for Dr. Peerwani. He wants to give you the guided tour."

"Oh, come *on!*" I said under my breath. After all, we'd been driving all night and we were eager to get started. Later, though, I'd come to appreciate Dr. Peerwani's caution. He knew that once we stepped into his lab, we'd be expected to jump in immediately and assist with the autopsies, and he wanted us to have at least a brief orientation before the relentless work began. Besides, this was his "shop," and we were here at his request. We needed to learn how things were done on his watch—and he wanted our absorption into his team to be as smooth as possible.

We had seen Dr. Peerwani on television almost every day, so when the darkly handsome Middle Eastern man in his starched white lab coat came through the door, we all stood in an instinctive gesture of respect. The doctor nodded and smiled but never broke stride as he signaled us to follow him into the inner sanctum of the morgue.

We hurried to keep up as Dr. Peerwani took us through the building, barely pausing to toss out a few brief words of introduction to the key people we'd be working with. As he identified various areas of the morgue, I tried to memorize every one of his quick, soft words, which held only a trace of a British-influenced accent. The building was like a maze and I worried that I'd never be able to find my way. But gradually a pattern started to emerge.

First came the "office areas," the ones where paperwork and research were done. At this early hour, workers were just beginning to fill these halls, turning on lights and opening doors in the staff's personal offices, library, and conference room. Here I saw furniture worthy of a well-heeled law firm, along with lush carpeting, large windows, and soft lighting fixtures. I even heard classical music seeping from under one closed office door. Office workers wore the standard professional suits and dresses.

Then, as we traveled deeper into the inner sanctum, the atmosphere changed along with the decor, as if we were following a photographer's gray scale from light to dark. Suddenly the big windows were gone, the carpet changed to tile flooring, and the institutional fluorescent lights hummed and flickered. Now we were in the lab, where forensics experts were just clocking in, busily covering their T-shirts and blue jeans with white lab coats. These people were getting ready to receive the vials of blood, tissue samples, and bits of trace evidence that would be taken from the bodies waiting for us downstairs, in the autopsy suite.

As we rushed downstairs, the uniform changed once again—the autopsy workers all wore light-blue surgical scrubs. Suddenly Dr. Peerwani stopped in mid-stride and we skidded to a halt, stacking up behind him. He turned and glanced at the three of us, then set off in another direction.

"Go change into scrubs before we go any farther," he said, nodding in the direction of two well-marked bathrooms. Theresa and I found ourselves in a large room that looked like a health club locker room— large lockers lining one wall, shower stalls and toilet cubicles in the back. Tall shelves stacked with light-blue surgical scrubs in several sizes stood right inside the door. We quickly took off our jeans and T-shirts and slipped on the scrubs over our underwear. Back in the hall, we now resembled the other workers we encountered as we continued our tour, except that these other people wore turtlenecks, thermal underwear, and heavy socks under their gear. And for good reason: As we got closer and closer to the autopsy suite, the air got colder—and the smell got stronger.

I will never forget that smell. Nothing I had ever experienced—in the operating room, on the Body Farm, on the few cases I had worked— even came close to this overpowering aroma. The nauseating smell of burned flesh—which I'd never really gotten used to—was now enhanced by the rancid odor of kerosene and the acrid scent of gunpowder. And pervading it all was the putrid smell of decomposing bodies.

Bill, Theresa, and I rolled our eyes and glanced at each other. As Dr. Peerwani flung open the double doors of the autopsy suite, we were sure we'd see burned and rotting corpses stacked floor to ceiling. What else could explain that overpowering smell?

Nope. Nothing. At this early hour, the morgue was empty. Four or five large stainless steel autopsy sinks lined the walls, and a cabinet full of rubber gloves, face masks, and other protective gear stood just inside the door. I noticed that the floors were scrubbed clean, the sinks were shiny, and just a few lights were on. I began to understand that the smells from a mass fatality seep into microscopic pores of the floor, ceiling, and walls. Water can flush away the visible evidence of death—but not the odors. They linger for a long, long time.

Dr. Peerwani was about to lead us into the adjoining x-ray room when he suddenly glanced at his watch and again broke off in mid-sentence. "Come on," he said once more, and the three of us found ourselves almost sprinting to keep up with him as he headed back to the conference room, where investigators were gathering for the seven-thirty a.m. briefing.

I knew how urgent it was to identify the bodies as soon as possible— bereaved families were waiting for the news, government officials were taking enormous amounts of political heat, and FBI investigators were still trying to determine what had really happened in the compound. So I didn't quite see why precious time was being taken out of the workday for a meeting.

Now, of course, I know that such briefings are standard protocol in any mass fatality, in which numerous agencies and large numbers of personnel are all working together at top speed. Everyone needs to be kept aware of the investigation as a whole, and it's important to have a time when the inevitable problems can be discussed and, hopefully, solved. Maybe a backlog in the x-ray department can be solved by pathologists being more selective in the views they request. Perhaps new phone lines need to be installed so that investigators can contact family members more easily. Or maybe more investigators are needed at the crime scene than in the morgue, requiring a reassignment of duty stations. It's also important, in a situation where so much is going on and rumors are flying madly, to keep the whole group informed with daily progress reports. It's good to start each day with a clear statement of where you are, what's not working yet, and what you hope to accomplish.

This day I saw yet another reason for a daily briefing: It gives the players on a very large team a chance to meet. Of the thirty or so people who filled the room, most had not even known each other, let alone worked together, before April 19. After only a week, though, they seemed very well acquainted, with Bill, Theresa, and I being the only newcomers. Then, to our surprise, we heard Dr. Peerwani saying our names.

"They're three forensic anthropologists just in from Tennessee," he explained, "and we're going to team them up with the forensic pathologists in the morgue to help separate and identify the skeletal material." Faces around the room nodded and smiled, and we smiled back gratefully.

I now know that many M.E.'s offices go along for years handling deaths in their own communities with no need for the specialized skills that my discipline can provide. Not until there's a mass fatality might they need some outside help. But if the M.E. doesn't quite know what forensic anthropologists do, it can be hard to coordinate the two disciplines.

Luckily, the Tarrant County M.E.'s office had an anthropologist on staff already, Max Houck. Max's primary job was as a trace-evidence analyst—someone who analyzes the tiny bits of evidence found at a crime scene, such as the hairs or paint particles left on a victim's clothes. But he had anthropological training, too, which meant that the pathologists in his office were used to teaming up with folks like us. Later, when I'd worked more mass fatalities, I'd realize what a huge difference that made. Max had given his colleagues a good idea of what they might expect from us, even though he wasn't at the briefing today—he was spending every possible minute out at the crime scene, locating and sorting the human remains.

Although I never worked the scene at Waco, I later learned what was involved in Max's assignment. In a fire like the one at Waco, there is a hierarchy of damage. Some victims emerge charred but relatively intact. Maybe their bodies were located on the periphery, or perhaps their remains were shielded from the inferno by falling walls, furniture, or even other bodies. Other victims have been reduced to fragments and body parts, which may have been scattered over a relatively wide area and mixed in with pieces from other people. The piles of charred torsos, the commingled arms, legs, and skull fragments, can be impossible to sort out completely at the scene, though Max and his team of Texas Rangers and medical investigators were certainly doing their best. Eventually, though, they simply had to bag and tag the remains they found, accepting that we at the morgue were going to get some body bags filled with the remains from several different people, all fused together from the heat of the fire. Or we might get a bag that held only the remnants of a hand, or perhaps a tiny T-shirt wrapped around a charred piece of skin and a baby bottle. Maybe we'd be able to match those fragments with pieces that came in other bags. Or maybe not.

Max and his team had worked out a system for keeping track of where each bag of remains was found. They'd created a crime scene diagram that enabled them to give each body bag its own number, showing us where the parts were found. We had a huge copy of this diagram posted prominently in a hallway next to the morgue, the body bag numbers marked out in red and the entire area sectioned off with an alphabetized grid. Knowing which body parts were found where could help pathologists and other investigators try to piece together exactly what had happened before, during, and after the fire— information that might be crucial at trial. And the diagram gave those of us in the morgue some common standard with which to begin the identification process. True, body parts might be blown across the site, with one person's hands in sector A and their feet in sector D; but, by and large, most people's remains tended to stay within a single sector. At least this way, we had a fighting chance of reuniting fragmented parts with their original owner, especially if someone had found a nearby torso or skull that we could identify. Hopefully, by the end of the investigation, every number would have a name.

As I worked other mass fatalities, I came to learn that each incident has its own unique problems of victim identification. In high-impact plane crashes, for instance, authorities have a reliable list of the presumed dead. Yes, you've got human tissues that are fragmented, commingled, and scattered, but at least you know who they're all supposed to belong to. When an office building collapses or goes up in flames, on the other hand, you're less certain of who might have been inside, but you can try to find people's identifying documents, such as driver's licenses, or hope that some of the victims were wearing jewelry or clothing that a spouse or parent will remember from that morning.

Here at Waco we had none of those clues. The list of the compound's residents was incomplete and in some cases had been intentionally obscured by the victims themselves, who included runaways, foreign nationals using false names, and U.S. citizens who had changed their names to conform to the sect's beliefs. And because they'd all been shut up together for days, no one on the outside had any idea of what they were wearing. Branch Davidians didn't carry wallets with IDs, nor did they indulge in materialistic practices like wearing jewelry (except a few pieces bearing the Star of David, which Koresh bestowed on some of his favorites). No one even knew exactly how many people had lived in the compound—but somehow the unique team of experts that had been assembled here would have to come up with a list of names.

That team—*my* team—had now made its way back to the morgue, and the previously quiet but smelly room seemed to be coming to life. I stood and watched from the sidelines as workers opened more doors into adjoining rooms. The door to the x-ray room featured the magenta trefoil—the international symbol for nuclear radiation— while a bright red light glowed above the door. "Do not enter when red light is on," warned a large sign. Another room was set aside for the dental identification team and still another for the fingerprint specialists. At the moment, though, the whole team was milling around the cabinet near the entrance to the main suite, climbing into their protective gear.

No one had time to tell me what to do, so I kept an eye on the seasoned staff and imitated them, thrusting my arms into a heavy cotton surgical gown so that the dangling strips of cloth would tie in the back. Then I grabbed a yellow surgical mask that I also tied in back, pulling it tightly over my mouth and nose. It didn't shut out the smell, but it did reassure me that I wouldn't be inhaling any stray spatters of blood. Next, I reached into a box and pulled out a one-size-fits-all pair of paper booties, which I slipped over my sneakers like a pair of galoshes. Another box held thin paper head covers, elasticized like shower caps, so I could tuck my hair underneath.

Theresa glanced over at me and laughed. "This is like striptease in reverse."

Her joke broke the tension, connecting us with the other workers. We all looked at one another and chuckled, and some of the bolder women began to wave their gear over their heads, doing a quick bump and grind before covering up every bit of exposed flesh. Getting a victim's blood on you was no joke. But it helped to laugh at ourselves.

I went on to don my face shield, a flat piece of thin plastic about twelve inches square, attached at the top to a layer of foam padding designed to fit gently against my forehead. I pulled a strip of elastic up over the back of my head, so that the plastic shield completely covered my face while the top circled my head like the old-fashioned stereotype of a Hollywood Indian's headband. I wished there was something I could put on to cover up the smell, but nothing I've found has ever really worked.

Last but not least came the coverings for our hands. Each of us was issued a pair of cut-proof gloves made from finely woven wire that resembled a miniature version of medieval chain-mail armor. Our supervisors warned us that broken glass and shards of metal were mixed in with the remains. Clumsy as they were, these devices would prevent injuries and the spread of infection through cuts. Thick rubber gloves went on over this armor for yet another layer of protection.

Covered from head to toe with cloth, plastic, paper, and chain mail, all we could see of each other was our eyes. We were finally ready to get down to work.

Someone snapped a few switches and all the lights came on as the huge exhaust fans roared into gear. Autopsy technicians—sometimes called "deaners" for no reason that I could ever tell—began wheeling gurneys into the room. Unlike the gurneys I'd seen in hospitals, these were asymmetrical, one end slightly higher than the other. On each gurney rode a black body bag with a large red number spray-painted on it. "MC-23," for example, was the twenty-third bag of remains recovered at Mount Carmel. The spray paint was an efficient—and waterproof—way to mark the bag boldly.

Each autopsy workstation was about ten feet long and three feet deep, with a large stainless steel sink flanked on both sides by elevated countertops. Each sink had three spigots connecting to a spray nozzle, a rubber hose, and a gooseneck faucet, giving us the maximum range of options for washing away the blood and gore. The whole unit rose to meet a three-foot-high backsplash equipped with lights, while the sink itself opened into the maw of a huge garbage disposal unit.

Two large steel rings in front of each sink lined up perfectly with the two large hooks at the end of each gurney. As the technicians wheeled the gurneys up to the sinks, they slipped the hooks into the rings and then used their feet to flip the locks at each of the gurney's four wheels. Now the gurney was part of our workstation. Each gurney had a two-inch hole in its lower end, sealed with a big black rubber stopper. This end now extended well over the lip of the sink, allowing us to uncork the gurney and drain fluids or rinse water down into the sink. The body bags were often simply left on the gurneys, so that we could roll them to another part of the lab without ever disturbing the remains.

Bill joined Dr. Gary Sissler, Theresa went to work with Dr. Peerwani, and I became a part of Dr. Charles Harvey's team. Dr. Harvey appeared to be in his fifties, a little shorter than I, but better nourished. He moved quickly and with purpose, immediately handing me a rectangular blue pan that looked for all the world like my own kitchen dishpan, though this one was filled with bloody remains. I immediately recognized them as pieces of burned skull mixed into a grapefruit-sized wad of baked blood and brains.

"Something just isn't right here," Dr. Harvey said, looking over my shoulder into the pan. "We originally thought all these people died from the fire. But this woman doesn't seem to have been burned all that badly. Her body was relatively intact and there was no soot in her airway."

I nodded. Usually, fire victims die from a rapid buildup of carbon monoxide while choking on the smoke. But this one had died *before* she'd had a chance to inhale anything harmful. Why?

"There's another thing," Dr. Harvey went on. "Investigators didn't see any evidence that any building debris had fallen on top of her—and yet her skull was in pieces. If it didn't get smashed in the crash or burned by the fire, what broke it?"

I looked down uncertainly at the charred remains. They held a secret that I had suddenly become responsible for discovering.

"I'll be anxious to see what you can do with this," Dr. Harvey said brusquely, and he went quickly back to his own new victim.

I stood uncertainly for a moment in the midst of the morgue traffic. Everyone seemed to be moving purposefully to his or her assigned task, but where was I supposed to work? Dr. Harvey's autopsy area was already filled to capacity with technicians, and stacks of instruments covered every horizontal surface. Finally I took the bucket over to a somewhat isolated white porcelain sink tucked into one corner of the morgue, checking to make sure it wasn't a "clean" sink—one of those closely guarded by safety watchdogs and reserved for hand-washing—before gingerly lifting out some of the pieces. I'd done this before, but never in this lab, surrounded with strangers, burdened by the knowledge that I was now part of a history-making event. I took a deep breath, forcing my mind to focus on the evidence I held and, as so often happens, my hands took on a life of their own, moving instinctively to tease the bone away from the brain.

It was the bones that caught my interest. The brain and other soft tissue had been essentially destroyed by the fire and the past week's process of decomposition. But the sturdy bones held secrets that I might decipher if I could just get the "squishy stuff" out of the way.

It was simple at first to grasp the largest pieces of the broken skull and pull them away from what was left of the brain. After I had scraped away the last of the baked blood and soft tissue from these large pieces, I washed them in a pan of hot soapy water, then set them aside on a blue towel to dry. The whole process was a little like doing the dishes after a particularly messy meal.

My goal was to reassemble the skull—only then could I read the story of the young woman's death—but in order to recover every single bone fragment, I had to pull the brain apart piece by piece, as if I were breaking off chunks of bread dough, my double-gloved fingers carefully probing the bloody tissue, seeking the bits of bone that were embedded within. As I extracted and then washed the smaller pieces, blood and dirty water splashed onto my chest and face shield and, to make matters worse, the occasional fly would land on me and crawl around. I soon discovered that if I tried to flick off the insect with my messy rubber gloves, I would spread more blood and gore to the spot where, before, only a little fly had left its tracks. So I did my best to ignore the flies and blood spatter that now covered not only my body but my face shield as well, a pockmarked pattern of black and red that left me feeling like I was looking through an insect-spattered windshield—without the wipers.

Then I began to discern the pattern that was gradually emerging in the skull fragments, and suddenly my discomfort vanished. Even at this early stage, I could see that these fractures were caused by something other than the fire, just as Dr. Harvey had suggested. But because of my anthropological training, I was able to see something in the bones that I recognized, though I could hardly believe my eyes. There was only one explanation for the way this woman's skull had shattered— but nothing I had heard in any of the news coverage or at this morning's briefing supported what I thought I saw.

My first impulse was to run over to Dr. Harvey and share my suspicions with him. But common sense and a sense of self-preservation prevailed. I'd had one too many run-ins with grad-school professors who'd taken me to task for "theorizing ahead of the facts." No, I'd gather every scrap of evidence I could before presenting Dr. Harvey with what I intuitively knew to be the truth.

So I removed the last morsel of goo from the skull bones before starting to dry each one with a paper towel. I knew that the next step was to glue the skull pieces together—that way, we could see the skull as it had been in life, and what I had discovered would be fully revealed. But the edges of the bones had to be entirely dry before the glue would stick and they were still soaking wet from their bath. I looked at them impatiently—maybe if I toweled them off?

One of the autopsy technicians must have seen me clumsily rubbing a few scraps of paper towel over the bones, because she suddenly tapped me on the shoulder. I turned around to see that she was holding a hair dryer in her gloved hand. She, too, was wearing a protective surgical mask, but I could tell by the crinkle at the corners of her eyes that she was smiling broadly underneath. I'm sure my eyes crinkled too as I smiled and took the dryer. In just a few minutes, I started gluing my bones back together.

Here is where Bill Bass's relentless pursuit of perfection paid off. Any other teacher might have allowed me to leave his class unsure of how to identify and reposition tiny random fragments. But thanks to Dr. Bass's insistence on detail, I could read the subtle variations in the contour of the bone and discern the delicate three-dimensional pattern of veins imprinted on some inside surfaces of the skull—clues that showed me at a glance which bones went where. As I had already done in my Tennessee murder cases, I started to glue the broken pieces together, edge to edge, just the way you'd piece together a broken vase.

Before too long the original shape of the woman's skull emerged: first her forehead, then her eye sockets, then the holes for the hearing mechanism and spinal cord. And then, as I placed two large matching pieces together, I saw exactly what I had expected to see, the evidence that I was longing to share with Dr. Harvey: a neat round hole with beveled edges in a place where the bone should have been smooth and solid. The hole's outside edge was surrounded by a ring by of black soot, also a significant clue. Dr. Harvey's first guess had been right.

Neither the fire nor the falling walls had shattered this woman's skull. She died because someone had held a gun up to her head and pulled the trigger.

The black soot told me how close the gun had been. You only get that sort of "gunpowder tattoo" when the gun's muzzle is close to the victim's head. I could see where the bullet had pierced the skull, too, breaking out a plug of bone as it forced its way through the skull's three primary layers—the smooth outer ectocranium, the inner endocranium, and the spongy bone sandwiched in between. As usually happens with entrance gunshot wounds to the skull, the entire three-layer bone plug had broken away at a slight angle, leaving a cone-shaped hole, sort of like the round window of a jet airplane, with the inside circumference of the hole larger than the outside edge.

Sometimes a bullet will also create an exit wound. That too leaves a beveled hole, but in the opposite direction, with the outside edge larger than the hole inside the skull. I didn't see that here, which meant that, theoretically, the bullet was still lodged in the woman's brain. But I hadn't found any trace of it, though I'd just squished through every square inch of brain matter, feeling for bone fragments. Was there a bullet or wasn't there?

I took a closer look at the skull. I could see that it was missing several fragments, probably pieces that the shot had blown away. Most likely, the exit wound was marked out on one of these missing pieces.

Now it was time to approach Dr. Harvey and ask him to examine my rebuilt skull. When I tentatively approached him, he stepped away from his own case without a word, businesslike but exhausted. I offered up the skull in its plastic pan like some weird project for art class, and he lifted the skull gently with both hands, slowly turning it around.

I heard his short, sharp intake of breath. The next thing I knew, he was dashing out of the room, taking the skull with him.

Standing there, still holding the blue pan in front of me, I glanced over to the team at the next autopsy station. They had just opened a body bag that contained hundreds of broken and burned bone fragments.

"You're an anthropologist, aren't you?" asked a male voice from behind one of the anonymous masks. I nodded and walked over to their gurney. "We could use you here," said the same muffled voice. And that's how it started. Two weeks of seemingly endless hopscotch in which I moved from task to task, helping out wherever I could.

Sometimes I would arrange groups of bones in anatomical order, separating the burned and fragmented tibias, fibulas, scapulas, hoping that a count of similar bones—two right femurs, for example—would help me determine just how many people's parts were in that pile. Or I might be asked to dissect someone's pelvic bones, examining the joints in a quest to determine the person's age. Most of the time, though, I was cleaning up skull fragments and gluing them back together, just as I'd done on that first case. Little did I know that the gunshot wound I'd found had been just the tip of the iceberg.

Besides the regular seven-thirty a.m. briefing, we also attended five p.m. sessions, when the medical personnel and FBI investigators gathered to share our findings for the day. On this first day, I was exhausted and happy to shed my protective gear, which by now was covered with a dense pattern of blood splotches, charcoal smears, some goo that was better left unidentified, and my own sweat. And I hadn't seen Bill and Theresa since Dr. Harvey had taken my arm that morning. I was anxious to compare notes, so I got back into my street clothes as quickly as possible and headed down the hall to join my friends. We barely had time to exchange greetings, though, before it was time to pour into the conference room. We three novices slipped into chairs against the back wall, just as the pathologists and federal agents took their seats around the conference table in the room's center.

As always, Dr. Peerwani opened the meeting, beginning today with a mundane list of the day's case numbers and a rundown of some positive IDs. He relayed a progress report from the scene and thanked everybody for the day's efforts. Then he yielded the floor to Dr. Harvey.

"I have some startling news to report," Dr. Harvey began. Bill, Theresa, and I leaned forward, wondering what he was about to say. "It concerns a woman found at the scene. Although her remains were burned, she didn't die from the fire. She died from a contact gunshot wound to the head."

Oh, my God, I thought. That's our victim, the one whose gunshot wound I found.

No one uttered a sound. They just looked at one another, some folks nodding their heads, others raising their hands to massage their aching temples. Still others had already begun furiously scribbling in their notebooks and, behind me, someone started tapping the keyboard of a laptop computer.

I later learned that our discovery had not been totally unexpected. Evidence from some of the earlier autopsies had suggested that at least some victims could not possibly have died from the fire, which was why Dr. Harvey had wanted me to examine the skull in the first place. Like others on the team, he had begun to suspect that at least some Davidians had been executed or had committed suicide before the smoke and flames reached their bodies. Today's discovery was the turning point, though—irrefutable proof that one of the victims had actually been killed by a contact wound to the skull.

Suddenly, the entire investigation was changing before my eyes. No longer was victim identification our sole mission. Every set of remains would now also have to be closely examined for even the most subtle signs of injury, and these findings had to be documented in detail. We would have to be able to distinguish between injuries incurred ante-mortem, perimortem, and postmortem—before, during, and after death. We would also have to try to determine the cause and manner of death—smoke inhalation? Flames? Being crushed by the building as it fell? Or had the victim been shot or stabbed or killed in some other way before the fire ever started? And then the victims would still have to be identified.

We were all dismissed from the debriefing with the assurance that a new protocol would be in place by morning, one that would hopefully address all of the issues that were just now bubbling to the surface. Meanwhile, Bill, Theresa, and I had to find a place to sleep. Before we'd left Knoxville, we'd prepared ourselves for the fact that if we couldn't find a cheap motel room that we could all afford to share, we'd have to camp out. Earlier that day, we'd started asking the other workers for suggestions and they'd all told us to talk to a tall white-haired man whom I'd seen circulating through the morgue throughout the day—Harold Elliott, chaplain for the Arlington Police Department.

Harold turned out to be our guardian angel. He immediately invited all three of us to stay with him and his wife, Norma, in their lovely home in the neighboring community of Arlington, Texas. We grate-fully accepted his offer, returning with him to what we soon came to see as our haven, a crucial refuge from the insanity we faced each day. Suddenly exhausted beyond belief, we managed to get a good night's sleep. Then, the next morning, it all began again.

●   ●   ●

Each day started the same way. A quick briefing, perhaps a reminder to make sure all the evidence was photographed or a warning not to speak to the press, and then I was off to change into my scrubs and get to work in the morgue. I greeted every day with anticipation and a sense of adventure. Each case was different and I was not only getting to make full use of my newfound forensic anthropology skills, but I was also absorbing reams of new information about mass fatalities.

I think what surprised me most was the degree of order hidden within the chaos. The numbered body bags, arriving fresh from the scene, were entered into a log, then stored in the cooler. When we were ready to work with them, they'd be pulled out, one at a time, and loaded onto gurneys, beginning their journey through an assembly-line system of analysis.

The sequence might vary, depending on what was in the body bag, but there was an established procedure for every type of situation. Pho-tography was always first. Documenting the evidence as it arrived from the scene was critical—especially now that we knew that this incident might not be just a horrible accident. The rumors of suicide and exe-cution were only now reaching the public, and the conspiracy theorists and reporters were having a field day. Speculation abounded. Had the FBI's hostage rescue teams killed the Davidians, peppering them with bullets as they tried to escape the flames? Or perhaps, as one particularly ugly rumor suggested, the angry FBI agents had pumped the dead bodies full of bullets, in some sort of bizarre battlefield revenge for their fallen ATF comrades.

Probably none of us would ever know exactly what had happened inside the compound. But our work would establish the best possible scientific foundation for interpreting the available evidence. Clearly, this case was going to trial, and there would probably be other legal inquiries as well. Maintaining the integrity of the evidence that was gathered—and keeping distortions out of the press—was crucial. So a single photographer, Chip Clark, was assigned to take all morgue photographs, while no one else was allowed to go anywhere near a camera. The investigators knew that Chip could be trusted: He worked at the Smithsonian Institution, which made him a federal employee, and he was fully aware of the protocols necessary for documenting evidence that would stand up in court.

Chip was charged with taking several different kinds of photographs. First, he recorded the initial appearance of each body bag's contents, which preserved a useful overview of the situation. Even more critical, though, was the documentation of particular images that might help tell the story of what had happened inside the compound. A picture of a burned hand encircled in a plastic wristwatch that had melted onto a clip of machine-gun ammunition was pretty telling evidence that hand and ammunition had been in intimate contact during the fire. A gas mask still stuck to the front of a child's face suggested that the child had been alive when the tear gas began to enter the compound. A unique piece of jewelry curled around the neck of a victim could be a crucial means of identification. The burned-off hand of a tiny child grasped in the hand of an adult female was a heart-wrenching record of these people's last moments—a detail that either prosecution or defense might incorporate into their stories about what had happened on April 19. Last but not least, Chip's photos gave us a permanent record of the medical evidence as we continued to search for the truth of that fatal day.

After photography came analysis. A pathologist or anthropologist had already opened the body bag for Chip to take his snapshots. Then the scientists examined the remains while dictating their findings out loud. A scribe took quick written notes, which a secretary would eventually transcribe into a computer file.

Without disturbing the tissues too much, the pathologist or anthropologist would start by trying to determine the sex, race, and approximate age of the victim. This was often not possible during the initial exam, though, because of the destruction and disarray of the remains. So this initial report might only describe the condition of the bag's contents, the degree of burning, and some general observations, such as whether the bag contained a large section of torso or just a few scraps of unrecognizable tissue.

On to the x-ray room. In some mass-fatality incidents, x-rays were left for later in the process, as they are usually used to determine such questions as whether the victim had old, healed fractures or perhaps a titanium hip replacement—ultimately useful for identification, but hardly the first priority here. What *was* a priority was making sure that these body bags were free of any unexploded ordnance, such as a hand grenade or another explosive. X-rays could also tell us whether any bullets or bullet fragments were hidden in the tissues, so that during the autopsy these could be located, documented, and removed.

Sometimes, too, these preliminary x-rays might reveal evidence of surgical hardware, such as a pacemaker. If so, the next step was to dissect such devices free from the surrounding body so that we could look for a serial number. Hopefully someone would find a matching number somewhere in the medical records of some victim on our (unreliable) list. Technicians also looked out for pins, screws, and plates used to repair fractures. Maybe we could find an x-ray or medical record documenting the fracture and its repair, enabling a positive ID.

If the body part in question held teeth, the dental identification specialists hurried over to take a quick look and make some notes. These amazing experts could tease secrets from even the smallest piece of dental enamel or burned tooth root—indeed, more than half of the victims at Waco were identified through dental comparisons. The trick here, as with the fingerprints, was finding a matching record. Luckily, many (though not all) of the adults at Waco had dental records on file, so after this quick initial survey, the dentists could start right in searching their files for a possible match. They'd get more time to examine the teeth after the autopsy.

Meanwhile, every moment that the conference room wasn't being used for briefings, investigators were constantly on the phone there, beseeching family members, dentists, and doctors around the world to send any and all records to Fort Worth. The fingerprint experts were going through a similar process—taking what prints they could find and then searching madly for a match. True, lots of the hands had been pretty badly burned, leaving very little skin from which to lift a print. But those FBI experts could sometimes work magic, managing somehow to pull prints from even the most charred fragments of tissue.

Of course, the most heroic print-lifting might produce disappointing results since, TV drama to the contrary, most people's prints aren't on file. There is a central computerized database that compares fingerprints and spits out IDs at the push of a button, but you soon find out that it doesn't cover most of the prints you're looking for—it only includes people with criminal records, and most mass-fatality victims don't have those.

Again, the protocol differs depending on the type of mass fatality. In a plane wreck, with a list of known victims, you can ask employers if they have their staff's prints on file. Or if you know that Jane Doe was on the plane, you can ask her husband to let you lift matching prints from her bathroom mirror or her can of hairspray. But at Waco, we had neither a reliable list of names nor very many printable hands. That put more pressure on the rest of us to try to take up the slack.

Investigators had responded by turning one end of the conference room into a command center dedicated to gathering information on the men, women, and children who had died. Men and women were constantly talking on the phone, ripping paper from the fax, making multiple copies of documents, and scrutinizing computer screens in a frantic effort to keep up with all the information that was pouring in. Little by little they filled out vital information on the growing list of names: age, race, sex, height, weight, eye color, hair color and length. If they could, the staff added other identifying details: prior injuries, surgeries, scars, tattoos. Authorities were holding in reserve the most tedious and time-consuming ID method of them all: the then relatively new science of mitochondrial DNA analysis. In the end, DNA told the story for many of our victims, but in the interests of speed and efficiency, we had to start with the more traditional methods, especially since DNA testing was then a complicated process that involved a number of steps taking anywhere from two weeks to more than a year.

Back in the morgue, the bags kept coming and coming, a seemingly endless procession of human debris. We anthropologists were in constant demand to help with victim identification. If a body had been reduced to a charred torso, we tried to determine the victim's age, race, and sex by examining the bones. This could at least narrow down the possible list of matching names. By now investigators suspected that there had been fifty-five adults, five teenagers, and twenty-three children in the compound when it burned. By further dividing the list of victims into male/female and White/Black/Asian, we made it easier to match charred remains to the names on our list.

The children were the hardest to deal with—both scientifically and emotionally. Max and his team had found many of the children wrapped in blankets, unscathed by the fire. Apparently the Davidian adults had put the young ones in the "bunker" area of the compound. Then the walls collapsed, burying the children under several feet of ordnance, burned structural debris, and other bodies. By the time investigators dug down under the rubble, the children's bodies had already begun to decay. At least they had been spared the worst ravages of the fire.

In order to locate the babies' tiny bones and teeth for analysis, we often had to search by touch. Each little corpse had been reduced to a rotting mass of flesh that revealed no secrets to even the most trained eye. The only way to learn anything was to feel around inside the mutilated body. You could usually find the skull bones pretty easily— they were relatively large, flat, and grouped together, even if they no longer held their characteristic globe shape. But in order to find the tiny pieces of still-growing bones and teeth, we had to start near the victim's head, manually compressing the cold, greasy, decomposed tissues until we felt the tiny, hard treasures we were seeking. Babies' backbones are still developing, with each vertebra composed of three irregularly shaped pieces resembling a set of toy jacks. When we examined shafts of the newborns' forearm bones, we found they were only slightly bigger than wooden matchsticks, while the bones of their fingers and toes were about the size of a grain of cooked rice. It may sound gruesome in description, but you'd be surprised how fast you get used to focusing on the physical details of the body, blocking out the reality of the little human who once inhabited it.

When we'd finally recovered what bones we could, we put the tiny pieces on top of a fine-mesh screen and rinsed them with hot soapy water. Then we had to try to identify the child, first trying to estimate the age and then perhaps the sex. The first time I worked on a child, the body still contained some identifiable soft tissue, so I was able to determine by looking at the genitals that I was working on a little girl. Later I'd get children who had been reduced to piles of burned bones—no soft tissue, nothing to tell me the sex. On an adult, that wouldn't matter: I can usually tell the sex of an adult arm or leg bone by measuring its size at the joint or by finding sex-marked features in a pelvis or in some morphologic feature such as muscle insertions—the places where muscles fit into the bone, which are generally more prominent in men. With young children, it's harder, since boys' and girls' bones pretty much resemble each other until puberty.

When I later worked on mass fatalities, I often used clothing to help determine gender, but I couldn't do that here. We had already been told that in the Davidians' communal compound, items of clothing were shared by all the children and essentially "unisex," with pretty much everyone wearing the same kinds of shorts and T-shirts. So now, since I was working on an unburned child, I turned to hair color and length to help with the ID. I cut off a lock of hair, washed it, and set it aside to dry. Later, I'd note its characteristics in that victim's permanent record, where hopefully it would narrow down the list of possible matches.

My job would have been far easier if this child had come to me with teeth still inside her mouth. As in most cases, though, the teeth had fallen out as the little body decomposed, and I had to feel around for them inside the cold, putrid, oatmeal-like soft tissues that had once surrounded her head and neck and filled her skull. As patiently as I could, I managed to retrieve fourteen teeth. I laid the teeth on top of a fine-mesh screen and rinsed them off with a stream of warm water from the sink before reinserting them into their sockets. I continued to pinch bones out of the goo, swishing them gently in a pan of warm soapy water and laying them out in anatomical order on a clean white sheet: first the skull fragments, then the neck bones, collarbones, shoulder blades, ribs, and so on toward the toes, until the little skeleton was complete.

Final analysis of the skeleton was left to one of the senior members of the forensic anthropology team, either Dr. Doug Ubelaker or Dr. Doug Owsley, both former students of Dr. Bass who now worked at the Smithsonian. The medical examiner's protocol required that only certain credentialed experts conduct the final analysis and sign their names to the official autopsy report. Fine with me. Still a graduate student, I was well aware of my limitations and was quite content to be a "worker bee."

So now, as I laid the final piece of the skeleton in place, I called for Chip to come photograph the skull's face with his Polaroid camera. Though I knew that taking Polaroids of the teeth was standard procedure, no one had ever actually explained to me exactly what the snaps were for. I later learned that during the siege, law enforcement negotiators had insisted that the adults in charge send out videotapes of the children in order to prove that they were well cared for and unharmed. Now FBI agents and dentists were analyzing the freeze-frame images from these same videotapes and comparing them to our "dental Polaroids." Since most of these children had never been to a dentist or doctor, this process of comparison was the only way to identify them, short of DNA analysis.

I was, frankly, proud of my burgeoning skill in assembling children's skeletons, and I soon learned to lean on that pride as a way to get through the long and grueling days. Satisfaction in a job well done filled me each time I called Chip over, refueling my energy for the next pile of bones.

One day, just as I was putting a child's last tiny tooth in place, I was asked to make a special trip to the conference room to deliver some autopsy findings. I walked into the conference room, my mind on the coffee break I was planning to take—and there on the screen was a freeze-frame image of a child who was strikingly similar to the one I had just been working on, a joyous little face, baring tiny teeth in a bright smile and waving "bye-bye" to the camera.

I was stunned. Tears welled up in my eyes, and my chest tightened. I looked away as quickly as I could, but it was too late. The image had burned itself into my retinas and suddenly my body was on its own recognizance, trembling and shaking in a way I didn't recognize.

I had to escape. I must have turned pale. I couldn't seem to move. Then, out of nowhere, a strong hand took hold of my elbow, and before I knew it I was in the inner sanctum of Dr. Peerwani's private office, as dazed as if I were lost in a sleepwalker's trance. When I finally became aware of my surroundings again, I discovered that I was sobbing uncontrollably in the arms of Harold Elliott, the strong and gentle police chaplain who was also my host.

Harold let me cry for what must have been about five minutes. Then he gently led me away—out of Dr. Peerwani's office, away from the morgue, the conference room, the videotape, away from the unforgettable image of that happy, smiling child whose little hand was still waving bye-bye in my mind.

"It's all right," Harold said softly as he ushered me into the front seat of his car. "Just let the feelings come."

I shook my head. How could I ever do my job with feelings like these?

Harold drove me to a nearby botanical garden, where for the first time in days I saw the midday sun and heard birds singing. When I was ready, I started to talk, and Harold listened. He was very good at listening.

"I just feel so helpless," I found myself saying. I hadn't known I felt this way—but then, I hadn't known I was ready to burst into tears, either. "All those people—all those *children*. Led like lambs to the slaughter, by people they trusted. And there's nothing I can do for them. It's too late."

"I know," Harold said quietly. "All you can do is what you're doing. But that doesn't mean it isn't hard."

Harold had spent most of his career as a chaplain for the Arlington Police Department. He was used to helping strong men deal with the despair and helplessness that seem to erupt routinely in situations where death and human destruction are served up on a daily basis. He knew that if I was to spend my life dealing with the dead, I had to learn to protect myself *from* the dead.

"You're no different from anyone else," he assured me. "If you didn't feel this way once in a while, you'd be a machine."

"But they all saw me," I said, mortified now by my loss of control in front of my colleagues. "What will they think?"

Harold shrugged. "They've all been there. The ones who have learned to deal with it will think exactly what I do—that you can't do this work without falling apart once in a while. The test comes in what you do next."

We sat for a while longer in the peaceful garden, the bright sun glinting off the shiny green grass at my feet. I realized how long it had been since I had seen any other light than the harsh white fluorescent bulbs in the morgue. How long it had been since I had smelled anything other than burnt bones and rotting flesh and smoke. I took a deep breath.

"All right," I said. "Let's go back."

Walking through the door of the morgue that afternoon was one of the hardest things I ever did. Maybe Harold understood what had happened to me—but these people were professionals. *They* hadn't lost control, and I couldn't expect them to be charitable about the fact that I had. And, indeed, some of my colleagues refused to look me in the eye as I walked in, pointedly turning away or simply ignoring my presence. The woman who had given me the hair dryer, though, made it a point to smile weakly and nod my way. So did the doctor who had pulled me into my first autopsy. He called me over now and handed me another blue plastic pan full of skull fragments. I took it quickly and gratefully slipped over to my favorite little sink. I picked out the pieces one by one, washing each one carefully in the warm soapy water. As I glued the skull back together, just as I had done on that very first day, a sense of déjà vu, settled over my shoulders as I watched yet another gunshot wound emerge.

•   •   •

Immersed as I was in the daily details of the investigation, it was easy to forget the big picture. But over the next week, I began to realize that we had gathered an increasing amount of evidence suggesting that many of the Branch Davidians had died in a mass murder-suicide. The half-dozen anthropologists on the project had found a total of eighteen gunshot wounds—eight definite, two probable, and eight "possible." The forensic pathologists examining the remaining soft tissue had found additional irrefutable evidence of gunshot injuries, bludgeoning, and at least one suspected stabbing. While the fragmented and incinerated remains would always hide the cause and manner of death for some victims, the evidence we uncovered was highly significant, and our supervisors meticulously documented even the tiniest details: carefully cataloguing the remains as they were recovered, conducting thorough autopsies on every victim, painstakingly reconstructing each shattered skull.

Ever since my first day, when I had managed to put that skull together in just a few hours, my colleagues had sought me out as the "skull lady," my own special niche in what we now called the "disassembly line." Practice makes perfect, and I could now pull apart and then put together these three-dimensional jigsaw puzzles in record time. It didn't always go as smoothly as it had the first time. Some of those skulls were extremely fragile, with large sections of bone blown away or burned up. But if I needed help holding pieces together while the glue dried or bridging the gaps with makeshift struts, Bill or Max was always right there by my side.

As our investigation drew to a close, we had established irrefutable evidence that more than one third of Waco's victims had sustained "non-heat-related trauma," which included contact or close-range gunshot wounds, shrapnel wounds, and blunt-force trauma—all before their bodies had ever felt the fire. We all believed that the true figure was a lot higher than one third, though without the evidence to prove it, the medical examiners duly listed many victims' cause and manner of death as "undetermined."

Members of the press continued—some still continue—to say that the Branch Davidians were all killed by the fire, but we knew that simply wasn't true. And though these reporters never hesitated to point an accusing finger at the federal government, they somehow still refuse to publicize the now-public autopsy findings, which prove conclusively that Waco ended in a mass murder-suicide orchestrated and carried out by the Davidians themselves.

As the days rolled on, our investigation developed a new focus: sect leader David Koresh. The charismatic figure had taken on a kind of near-mythic status, and there was even speculation that he and some of his henchmen had somehow escaped the inferno, fueled by a *National Examiner* "eyewitness report" of Koresh jumping into a getaway car at the end of a tunnel leading out of the compound. Unless we positively identified his remains, no one would ever be certain if Koresh lived or died. The last thing any of us wanted was for the self-styled messiah to earn some sort of mythic status that would inspire his cult to spring up again. And if he was by some chance alive, the FBI wanted him at the top of their Most Wanted list.

So, back in the lab, we were keeping a close watch for any remains that might be associated with Koresh. Our first break came on the afternoon of May 1, when pathologists began to examine body bag "MC-08." Our dentists had earlier obtained a model of the cult leader's teeth and they knew, almost by heart, what dental evidence they were looking for. They'd made it a matter of routine to check every body bag for Koresh's telltale stainless steel crown and missing premolar, and I'll never forget the sight of Rodney Crow, our chief forensic dentist, bending over MC-08 as we all held our breath.

Crow stood up slowly, straightening his back to the fullest. "That's him."

"Are you serious?" asked someone hidden behind a mask.

"I'm serious. That's him." A huge Cheshire-cat grin spread over Crow's face and then quickly disappeared. We had finally found David Koresh.

Koresh's postmortem exam the next morning followed the standard autopsy protocol, but given the high level of controversy surrounding his demise, a lot more people than usual made sure to check and double-check the evidence. Chip Clark, camera at the ready, never left Dr. Peerwani's side as the corpse was x-rayed, examined, and identified. It was standing room only around the gurney as we watched Dr. Crow make a detailed record of the dental evidence. Then Dr. Peerwani called me to his side as he began to sift through the burned debris and bones found near the victim's head.

"It looks like I may have a little job for you here, Emily," he said in a low voice. "I'd like you to go get ready to piece this one together just as soon as I've collected the fragments."

He refused to speculate about what I might find—and I too was finally learning not to "theorize ahead of the facts." Still, I had reconstructed enough skulls shattered by gunshot wounds in the past five days that I could readily recognize the same type of injury here.

However, "Yes, sir," was all I said. I backed off and signaled to Max Houck, who had finished at the crime scene and was now working with us in the morgue.

"This is going to be huge, Max," I muttered under my breath. "I think we should do this together. I know I'd feel a lot more secure if a second pair of hands and eyes was involved each step of the way."

Max nodded and we went over to the sink, laying out the toothbrushes, scissors, and knives we would need if we found remnants of tissue clinging to the bones. I filled my trusty blue plastic pan with warm soapy water, took off my double set of heavy protective gloves, and put on two pairs of thin surgical gloves instead. I was already a little nervous about doing this case, and I wanted all the manual dexterity I could muster.

Half an hour later, Dr. Peerwani had filled a metal tray with dozens of skull fragments, most of them burned, some no larger than a dime. He brought the tray over to our sink and ceremoniously handed it to me.

Naturally, there was a flurry of extra attention given to this all-important part of the autopsy. FBI agents, pathologists, and the other anthropologists jockeyed for better spectator angles, only to be nudged aside by Chip Clark, our intrepid photographer, who needed to get some preliminary photos before we started work. It was a little unnerving to have such close scrutiny as I delicately picked pieces of fragile bone from the tray, cleaned them off, and laid them out in some semblance of anatomical order—pieces from the face in one spot, bones from the back of the head in another, side pieces in a third.

Then, as often happens when I work, I forgot where I was, focusing only on finding each piece's proper place. Max and I made a good team, sharing our task wordlessly. Sometimes he could pick out a piece from the pile that matched the color of a piece I was holding. A few times we simultaneously picked up separate pieces whose fractured edges matched in shape or whose anatomical landmarks lined up. Once again, I thought of piecing together a three-dimensional jigsaw puzzle, though in this case huge sections of the puzzle were missing.

Nevertheless, by noon we were ready to start gluing the pieces together. On an ordinary day it would have been lunchtime, but we were both too engrossed to think of food. Instead, Max brought out the new two-part glue we had started using to reconstruct the skulls. It worked on wet items and hardened instantly, even expanding slightly to fill in gaps where necessary. It took two people to use it, though; one to hold the bone fragments together, the other to squeeze the applicator bottle. A tiny amount of watery liquid would dribble down into the crack between the bones, while the "gluer" quickly set down the bottle and picked up a small spritzer. Once the second element had been sprayed onto the skull—sometimes accompanied by a dramatic little puff of smoke—the chemical reaction was instant and irreversible. If the "bone handler" had remained immobile throughout the process, the bones were now permanently fused.

This painstaking process had to be repeated with each new matching fragment, so Max and I took turns holding and spraying. Even so, the strain of holding the bones perfectly still was nerve-wracking, and each of us found that after only a few minutes our fingers started to tremble or even to curl up with muscle cramps.

Word had reached the break room that we had started to glue Koresh's skull back together, and we were abruptly joined by a curious matinee audience who had suddenly agreed that this was indeed more important than lunch. Large portions of Koresh's frontal and left parietal bones were missing but, gradually, before all our eyes, the skull took shape in my hands and the gunshot wounds emerged.

Max and I were so focused, we didn't even realize that the room had become eerily quiet. The half-dozen men watching over our shoulders hadn't said a word since they spotted the first evidence of the gunshots, but I could hear some of them breathing, their mouths only inches from the back of my neck. Maybe it was their warm breath, or maybe it was just nerves, but when I put the last critical pieces in place, the hairs on the back of my neck started to tingle. Max's eyes met mine, and I saw his pupils dilate—an uncontrollable reaction signaling excitement and pleasure. I suspect that my eyes mirrored his, because I felt as if I were blushing, the blood pounding in my ears. I was sure the guys standing behind me could hear my heartbeat.

The spell was broken when the double doors flew open and Dr. Peerwani sailed into the room, the tails of his long white lab coat flapping in his wake.

"I just heard that you've found gunshot wounds in his head!"

"Yes, sir." Max and I spoke almost in unison.

"Show me, please, Miss Craig." Dr. Peerwani's good manners and respect for his workers never failed, even in this critical moment.

I picked up the skull and pointed to the semicircular hole in the middle of the forehead. It was beveled inward, surrounded with the sooty tattoo that was the earmark of a contact gunshot wound. Then I carefully turned the skull upside down so the doctor could see the exit wound. The bullet had left the lower part of the back of the skull, not too far from the spinal cord.

It was an unforgettable moment. We all stood in silence together, thinking back over the past weeks—all the remains we'd identified, the children we'd labored over, the death and destruction that Koresh had caused. We thought of the people whose remains had passed through our hands, the families who would never see their loved ones again. We thought of the horror of April 19, watching the flames flicker across our TV screens, and we thought of the rumors that had blared from those same TVs, the accusations that the FBI had murdered Koresh and his followers, the claims that the Bureau had set the fire that killed everyone. Now I held Koresh's skull in my hand for all of us to see, marked with the unmistakable evidence of the cult leader's death by an intimate hand. No FBI agent could ever have gotten close enough to Koresh to press a gun to his skull—and this beveled hole ringed with soot could only have been made by such a gun. Koresh was dead from a contact gunshot wound to the forehead, and we, together, had proven it.

Chip had been taking pictures throughout the reconstruction. Now he was hoping to get a good shot that would show the entrance and exit wounds at the same time. No camera could show both, however, no matter which way we turned the skull. I leaned over and whispered a suggestion to Max, who nodded in agreement. From our casual chitchat, he knew I was a certified medical illustrator, so when I offered to make drawings of the injuries—drawings that Dr. Peerwani could then use to describe his findings—Max readily agreed. Dr. Peerwani gave us his clearance right away, as did Dr. Doug Owsley, today's forensic-anthropology team leader.

Though I'd expected to draw only Koresh's head, Dr. Peerwani asked me to make drawings of his hip as well. While Max and I had been putting the skull together, our colleagues at the next table were examining his hip and lower spine. Spinal x-rays had matched x-rays taken by Koresh's chiropractor before the siege—one more proof that we had indeed found our man. Dr. Peerwani had also discovered that Koresh had a large, healing gunshot wound in his left innominate (hip) bone at the time he died, probably from the first shootout with ATF back in February. (Transcripts made from phone conversations and videotapes made during the siege had led investigators to this conclusion about Koresh's injury.) Chip had documented the hip bone with photographs, but Dr. Peerwani wanted a drawing as well. I was happy to oblige.

As I began my sketches, using the same sort of plain white paper and number 2 pencil that I'd used for Dr. Hughston, I couldn't help feeling that I had come full circle. I worked late into the night, making sketches of injuries in the rebuilt skull from four different angles, along with a view of the hole in Koresh's hip. These drawings became part of the autopsy report, which confirmed that Vernon Howell, a.k.a. David Koresh, had died from "massive craniocerebral trauma due to a contact gunshot wound to the mid forehead." Before the next day was over, facsimiles of my drawings had been sent to FBI director William Sessions—and to his boss, Attorney General Janet Reno.

The drawings were such a success that Dr. Peerwani quickly asked me to illustrate several more of the gunshot wounds that had been sustained by the victims. That was how I spent my last week at Fort Worth—cleaning bloody brains from the skulls, gluing the pieces back together, and documenting my findings. Given how my first day had gone, it seemed a fitting conclusion.

• • •

I turned a page in my professional life during those few weeks. Now more than ever, I saw forensic anthropology as a crucial way of finding out what had happened, helping investigators solve the riddles of the dead. But I had also stumbled upon the contradiction that would always mark my work. No matter how skilled or professional I might become, my elation at solving forensic problems would forever coexist with suppressed despair for the victims.

When I returned to the university, I threw myself into my final year's casework with a new urgency. I was now more determined than ever to find a full-time job doing exactly the kind of work I had done at Waco. To do that job well, I'd need to soak up every bit of knowledge in the few months of school that remained to me. After all, my on-the-job initiation at Waco had put me under the supervision of some of the most distinguished forensic anthropologists in the world. Once I graduated, I'd be on my own.

4

Crying Out for Justice

The dead cannot cry out for justice,
it is a duty of the living to do so for them.
— LOIS MCMASTER BUJOLD

T HE BLACK BLOWFLIES were so heavy and slow in the summer air
that I could knock them to the ground with my bare hand.
The two dead bodies over which they swarmed already
seethed with maggots, offspring of the flies that had gotten there several days before me. As I knelt beside the woman's body, sweat running
from my forehead and puddling inside my oversized glasses, I felt as
though someone had draped my shoulders with a hot, wet blanket.

The bodies lay only a few yards apart, so just by pacing back and
forth through the weeds I could see that each of them was at the same
stage of decay. They had both been killed at about the same time—not
too long ago, judging by the faintly lighter green of the grass peeking

out from underneath their bodies. If they'd been here more than a few days, the grass would have yellowed; if they'd been here longer than that, it would have died completely.

I was also fairly certain that someone had tossed these bodies here when they were already dead. Their arms and legs were in awkward disarray, and no nearby plants had been disrupted—no broken stems or wilted stalks to indicate a struggle. The lack of pooled or spattered blood on the grass also told me that the bodies had been put here after death, when blood remains within the body because there is no beating heart to force it out.

These two had not died gently. Their skulls had actually warped from the attacks they had sustained—a common occurrence with low-velocity blunt-force trauma, which can cause bone to literally bend before it breaks, never to return to its original shape. Only the murderer knew just how much force it had taken to do that, and to split the skulls into the pieces I saw here, but at least I could read part of these victims' story in the large gaps of missing bone and in the fracture lines that crisscrossed their caved-in skulls. I knew, too, that as they lay there, with their broken and bloody skulls, flies had chosen those warm, moist areas to lay their first eggs, and I could see their hatching larvae concentrated there now, busily consuming everything except hair, bones, and teeth.

A little more than a year had passed since I'd been at Waco, and this was the first case for which I was completely on my own. Just three working days ago, on July 1, I'd signed on as State Forensic Anthropologist, making me responsible for the analysis and identification of decomposed bodies and skeletal remains found anywhere in the Commonwealth of Kentucky. But even if I'd already worked a thousand cases, this would have been a tough one.

It started when a farmer had discovered the bodies of this woman and child in the tall grass at the edge of a fallow pasture somewhere near the close-knit town of Somerset, in Pulaski County. By the time I got to the scene, the sheriff's deputies had already identified the victims as a twenty-one-year-old woman and her four-year-old half-brother, last seen sitting on the steps of a neighborhood church on the afternoon of Sunday, just four days before. Obviously, they hadn't been murdered on the church steps—but where *had* they died? And when, and how? Obviously, the murderer had fractured their skulls—but had he shot them first? Beaten them to death? Or perhaps they had died by stabbing or even strangulation, the final beating merely an angry aftermath? If I could help investigators answer these questions, we might be able to answer the biggest question of all: Who killed them?

Coroner Alan Stringer had called me right after noon, asking me to come down to help with the crime scene investigation. Three days into the job, and I couldn't have found Somerset on a map—luckily, I was able to catch a ride with a couple of state police lab techs also assigned to the case. I didn't know any of the investigators yet, either, who were now standing behind me in a loose semicircle, safely away from the overwhelming smell. Sheriff Sam Catron stepped up and introduced himself, gallantly volunteering to assist with what he knew was going to be a difficult job. The good-natured mix of uniformed deputies and detectives in street clothes backed off just far enough to where they could watch my every move and see how I was going to work beside their fearless leader. I brushed ineffectually at the swarm of flies now buzzing around my head and wondered if the overwhelming smell would make me faint. It was time to collect samples of my old nemesis: maggots.

I started with the woman, whose skull bones peeped out from under a mass of dark, wet, maggot-filled hair. Normally, I'd gather maggots with a small spoon-like scoop, but I was so new to the job that I hadn't yet gotten my crime scene kit in order. Stifling a grimace, I reached into the maggot mass with my latex-gloved hand and pulled up a handful. As they writhed in my palm, I used my other hand to pick out a dozen long, plump ones and drop them into a little plastic cup, the kind doctors use to collect urine samples. My goal was to "freeze them in time"—to kill them while leaving their bodies intact—so that an entomologist could tell us just how old they were.

At school I'd killed maggots by filling my specimen jar with 70 percent isopropyl alcohol, but that was yet another item that was missing from my crime scene kit. Maybe if I covered them with scalding water?

"Okay, but where in the world am I going to find boiling hot water, way out here . . . ?" I had been literally thinking out loud during this whole process, talking through each one of my actions for the benefit of my colleagues. This was a technique I'd developed during my Tennessee casework, when I'd realized that, otherwise, my actions seemed meaningless at best, downright weird at worst. Besides, sharing my process gave others a chance to offer a helping hand.

Sure enough, one of the detectives called out, "What about the radiator in your van? Y'all just drove a hundred miles. It should still be plenty hot."

"What a brilliant idea!" I cocked my head at my fellow investigators, held out my cup of maggots, and smiled sweetly. "Can one of you please take care of this for me?"

I sat back on my heels and waited as the investigators shuffled their feet and looked sideways at each other. Finally, Deputy Coroner Tim Phelps sidled over and tentatively took the cup. He headed back to the van and I went back to picking maggots off the woman's body. From somewhere behind me, I heard the sound of a hood popping open and then Tim's agonized groan of disgust as he siphoned scalding water from the radiator over the writhing insects. I tried to hide my smirk.

Much to Tim's dismay, I wasn't finished. He watched me extract samples from the maggot mass churning in the woman's pubic area, then bravely made a second trip back to the van. I moved on to collect still more samples from the little boy, labeling each cup with the place on the body from which they'd been taken, along with the date, time, case number, and my initials.

To Tim's—and my—enormous relief, the maggot-collection part of my work was soon finished. Now it was time to take the temperature of the maggot mass itself, a task requiring the coroner's extra-long thermometer, the one he used to stick in the liver or rectum of recently dead bodies to find out how much they'd cooled off. If you slid the thermometer into the various maggot masses in the woman's and boy's bodies, you could document more information that might help determine time of death.

Next it was time to document the temperature and humidity of the air that enveloped the bodies—the same hot, sticky air that was making it so hard for me to breathe. The entomologist would eventually need this climatological data, so today and every day for a week the coroner or a deputy would have to return to this spot and document the temperature and humidity. The entomologist would then be able to look at the data and the maggots and work backward to figure out when the flies had first laid their eggs, when the maggots started feasting on the dead bodies—and when the bodies might have shown up in the field.

I went on to document the bodies' location, taking photos and making a quick sketch to remind me of their relationship to the surrounding scene. The sheriff's deputies were experts in this sort of procedure, so I left them to their more detailed sketches while I studied the two victims once more. Their postcranial area—everything from the neck on down—was still intact, which meant that any clues in these areas were the province of the forensic pathologist. Although there are some areas of overlap, pathologists usually deal with the soft tissues, while I deal with the hard ones—bones and teeth. If enough of the body is intact to permit a traditional autopsy, the pathologist conducts it, documenting the general appearance of the person and the internal organs, and collecting blood and tissue samples for analysis. If not enough soft tissue remains to yield any clues, then we rely on the bones, which I usually work on by myself. This division of labor—soft versus hard tissue—can be confusing to crime-show fans, since TV pathologists tend to appear as experts in all things; but in the forensic world, a person has usually either studied soft tissue and gotten an M.D. or has studied hard tissue and gotten an M.A. or a Ph.D. in anthropology. After all, no one can specialize in everything.

"Go ahead and bag them," I told the coroner now, knowing that his men would take the bodies to the morgue. Tomorrow the forensic pathologist and I would do an autopsy together—him focusing on the soft tissue, me concentrating on the bone.

The coroner and his deputy wrapped each body in a clean white sheet and placed it in an individual body bag. Until we got a positive ID, the bags were labeled John and Jane Doe.

As the coroner was zipping up the first bag, I moved to the soil where the little boy's head had lain. Luckily, I'd brought a hand trowel, which I now dragged across the soil and matted grass. Piece by piece, a little treasure trove emerged: brownish-gray fragments from his shattered skull, tiny teeth that had separated from the rest of his head during decomp, and small black tufts of hair that had fallen away as his scalp sloughed off. Sealing my collection in a small plastic bag, I quickly labeled it "from head area of child victim" and tucked it inside the boy's body bag. As the guys carried the bag to the coroner's van, I made a similar collection in the spot where the woman had decomposed.

The police and sheriff's men had finished documenting the scene and were now fanning out across the surrounding field, searching for any remaining evidence. I'd finished my work though, so I stripped off my gloves, tore open a package of disinfecting towelettes to wipe my dripping face and hands, and plumped myself down on a clean patch of grass to drink a bottle of cold spring water.

"Well, I'm sorry we had to meet under these circumstances, but I'm sure glad you came down here." Alan, the coroner, was sitting down beside me.

"Hey, a double homicide after three days on the job—I feel like I've just jumped into the deep end of the pool."

Alan laughed quietly and handed me a clipboard full of forms.

"You know, Alan," I said quickly, "this is my first case here in Kentucky. Think you could help me out with the paperwork?"

He grinned. "Don't worry, Doc, we got you covered." He began to leaf through the pages with me. We continued to talk about the case until Alan asked finally, "So you and Dr. Hunsaker will do the autopsy tomorrow?"

I nodded. "Yes, he and I had better work on this one side by side—if that's okay with you."

This was all old hat to Alan, but I was still getting used to the Kentucky procedure. Because Kentucky is such a large and rural state, every county has its own elected coroner, who serves as the primary death scene investigator after receiving special training in forensic death investigations. Elected coroners are not usually M.D.s, and even if they are, they don't do the autopsies. Instead, the coroner normally works the crime scene, sending any bodies that need autopsies to one of four regional state medical examiner's offices, where forensic pathologists who are M.D.s analyze the body further. The coroner has ultimate responsibility for his or her county, however, authorizing the pathologist to do the autopsy, receiving the final report and, ultimately, issuing the death certificate.

Sometimes the coroner also needs a bone specialist, in which case he or she calls me. I might come out to the crime scene, assist at the autopsy, or take the bones back to my lab in Frankfort. In this case, pathologist Dr. John Hunsaker would be analyzing the bodies' soft tissue while I tried to figure out what had happened to their skulls.

"Any thoughts so far?" Alan asked.

"Well, it's obvious their skulls were shattered," I said slowly. "But right now I can't tell just how. And I strongly suspect they were dumped here, not killed here." I was also fairly certain that the victims had died by blunt-force trauma—from being beaten, not shot or stabbed—but I wouldn't really know for sure until I'd had a chance to go back to my laboratory and rebuild the skulls. Since bones break in a fairly predictable manner, rebuilt skulls—or even skull fragments—can often help us figure out what caused the damage. At the very least, we might be able to rule out some potential weapons. Bullet wounds are pretty distinctive, but blunt-force trauma can also leave clues. The round end of a ball-peen hammer, for instance, often leaves a ball-shaped indentation, while a tire iron or the shaft of a golf club tends to leave a long narrow groove.

To get a true picture, though, you need to recover as many skull fragments as you can. Although in this case I'd found lots of loose skull pieces on the ground, I could see that several more fragments were still embedded in the congealed blood and decomposing brain tissue packed within the "brain case," the cranium. John and I would have to work out a carefully choreographed sequence in tomorrow's autopsy to make sure that neither of us damaged the other's evidence.

For both of us, the maggots were going to be both help and hindrance: a help because they'd enable us to narrow down the postmortem interval, or "time since death"; a hindrance because as long as there were maggots in the body, they'd continue to devour its flesh even if the coroner put the bodies in the morgue cooler.

A maggot mass can take on an astonishing life of its own once it gets established in a carcass. Thousands of maggots can accumulate in a dead victim's chest cavity or pelvis, sort of like a chicken carcass packed tight with lots of creamy overcooked rice. Then the maggots pull together into a cohesive group that churns and boils continually when the air temperature gets too cold for them, as individual maggots try desperately to reach the core for warmth, pushing their hapless neighbors to the periphery—only to be themselves pushed out of the way by yet more desperate maggots. At night or in the morgue cooler, the collective maggot metabolism can be as much as 10 degrees higher than the rest of the body's temperature, so when the body emerges from the fridge, you're likely to see a cloud of steam rising slowly from your homicide victim's collapsed and half-devoured chest.

"Put the bodies in the freezer, not the cooler," I told the men. Most maggots can survive those sub-zero temperatures, but at least the freezer's extreme cold would arrest their appetites and make them sluggish. Let's take every opportunity we humans have—the maggots will get their turn soon enough.

· · ·

The next day at autopsy, the victims' chest cavities were indeed packed tightly with maggots. For now, they were immobilized—stunned from the cold—but in less than an hour, they'd start to move again. John and I would have to hurry.

I was dressed in the usual blue-green scrubs, surgical gown, gloves, mask, and face shield. My gear protects me from everything but the smell, which always seems to soak right into my skin, my hair, my nose, even my taste buds. Menthol cream smeared under my nose doesn't seem to help, either—it just adds more noxious fumes to the mix. When I first started in this line of work, I thought someday I'd get used to it—but I haven't.

This would be a conventional autopsy, so I was only responsible for the teeth and skull bones. I'm always grateful for the "learning by touch" that Tyler and I had practiced in osteology class, given how many times I have to resort to compressing soft tissues manually in order to retrieve bone and teeth fragments, much as I'd done with the children at Waco. Skull fragments and teeth often filter down into the base of the skull, the neck, or even the victim's decomposing chest cavity, and then I have to grope around to find them, feeling through dark brownish-green tissues that resemble nothing so much as chocolate pudding into which someone has stirred a few cups of chunky vomit.

Meanwhile, the body is still home to tens of thousands of maggots, boiling up out of the chest cavity like suds overflowing from a washing machine. Someone once naïvely asked me why I couldn't simply remove the maggots before doing an autopsy, and all I could do was shake my head and chuckle. By the time we got rid of the maggots, there'd be nothing left of the body.

Still, the notion of fumigating a maggot-filled body is an appealing fantasy, because after my hands have been dipped in this cauldron of gore for a few minutes, the maggots start to climb up my sleeve, coated with a sticky mucus that allows them to cling to a number of different surfaces. Over my gloves and arms they crawl, migrating up toward my face, with its tempting facial openings. . . . I am so repulsed by their slow, determined journey that my reflexes often take over, causing me to flick my wrist and send several maggots hurling to the floor. That seems like a good place for them—until they start to wriggle off under the counters or climb up the leg of another lab worker or an unsuspecting med student who's come along to observe. So once those maggots hit the floor, you've simply got to step on them—even though stepping on an engorged adult maggot is like smashing a miniature grape. They pop—and their pus-colored innards smear over the floor, making yet another mess. To me there's no contest, though: better underfoot than on my face.

Over the years, I've developed a number of little tricks to cope with my maggot friends. I've learned to work quickly and to keep the autopsy room as cold as possible. That at least renders the maggots a little sluggish, giving us humans a slight but crucial advantage. Even more than the cold, maggots hate bright light, so whenever possible, I put a large black trash bag over a central portion of the body. After a while the maggots migrate underneath. Slowly I slip the bag down to the other end of the gurney, with many maggots following desperately along, leaving me to work in relative peace. It's nice to feel smarter than a maggot.

"Well, Emily, you're certainly starting off with a bang," John commented as we began today's autopsy. He looked like your stereotypical college professor—kind of handsome in a studious sort of way, tall and a bit stooped, with his glasses perpetually dangling from a cord around his neck. He always wore a soft brown Mr. Rogers sweater to ward off the chill in the morgue, and he puffed continually on a large wooden pipe to help kill the smell.

"I know," I said as he cut into the body and flipped a few maggots of his own onto the floor. "A double murder. Not bad for three days on the job."

"Don't forget to find some tenants for your 'maggot motel,' " he said with a grin. I knew he understood the science behind it, but I defy anyone to say "maggot motel" with a straight face. Since many maggot species look similar, the entomologist needs to see the adult flies, and so it was my lucky job to collect another dozen larvae from the body and raise them to adulthood. Although all of the pathologists know how to do this, they're even more squeamish than I am when it comes to maggots, so if I'm around, my colleagues are more than willing to pass this duty on to me whether or not it's a skeletal case. I use a simple milk carton with some dirt on the bottom and a small chunk of chicken liver wrapped loosely in aluminum foil. The maggots gorge themselves on the liver, then bury themselves in the dirt to pupate. One of the weirdest parts of my job is my nightly bed-check at the maggot motel, making sure my little charges are alive and well and have plenty to eat.

"I'll never get used to those things," I said now. "Hey, John, do me a favor, will you? Take a few more puffs of your pipe." The second-hand smoke covered the smell for me, too.

•   •   •

After John and I had finished the autopsy, I cleaned the skulls and skull fragments, submerging them into warm soapy water and scrubbing them clean with a toothbrush, just as I'd done at Waco. I left them to dry overnight and returned the next day to begin the laborious process of gluing the skulls back together.

In this case, all my questions centered on the skulls, but later I'd run into cases where I had to clean and examine every single bone in a body, searching for skeletal trauma or maybe evidence of an old injury to help me make an ID. This doesn't happen very often, maybe one case in five, but when it does, it's a real chore—messy, time-consuming, and smelly. It's something like deboning a rotten chicken though, of course, on a much larger scale. I use x-rays and photographs to help me figure out some way of working the bones free from the decomposing flesh without damaging them. After all, some of the bones might hold tiny cut marks or other evidence of a murderer's actions, and I don't want to leave my own trace evidence alongside of his.

If there's not too much flesh, I can usually pull the bones out of the soft tissue with a very tiny tweak, like twisting a stem off an apple. If I meet even the slightest resistance, though, I'll dissect the bones away with a small pair of blunt-tip, curve-bladed scissors. Again, my main concern is not to nick or cut any of the cartilage or bone. As I remove each bone from its fleshy casing, I place it on another gurney, aligning my collection in anatomical order. That way, I can do a skeletal inventory while I work, noting what's missing and checking each bone as I lay it into place—my first chance to look for breaks, bruises, or other anomalies that might offer us clues.

If the bones are still too fleshy to reveal their secrets, I'll take them to the corner of my lab that my colleagues jokingly call "Miss Em's kitchen." There I boil the bones gently, cooking off any remaining flesh in a process we call "thermal maceration."

Like any good cook, I have my system. I fill two Crock-Pots and a large covered roasting pan with water and some mild dish-washing detergent, which helps cut the grease. I like to have my pots full and ready to go before I even start recovering the bones, so I can drop everything into the water and turn on all the devices at the same time. That way, I know exactly how long each bone has cooked, and I can be certain nothing cooks too long. I make sure that the water heats up gradually, too, so that each bone can adjust to the heat.

I'm happy to report that thermal maceration will destroy even the most tenacious of maggots, including those which hide themselves deep within a bone's nerve and artery channels. If I'm in a particularly sadistic mood, I'll watch as the water heats up and the maggots swarm frantically out of their hiding places. They rise to the top of the steaming liquid, writhing momentarily on the greasy film that forms on the surface before they succumb to the heat. Occasionally some of the more athletic maggots even manage to scale the Crock-Pot's ceramic liner—only to sizzle and pop when they slide down the other side and land on the cooker's hot metal frame.

I hadn't had to boil any bones, but it had taken me several hours to reconstruct the skulls, working by myself and using simple household glue out of a tube. As I stood by my shiny morgue table, watching them dry—the large skull for the woman, the little one for the child—I felt a bitter satisfaction. My colleagues and I had collected a huge amount of evidence that might someday be used to convict a killer. Of course, I'm a scientist, and my focus is on the evidence, not the criminal or the crime. And even as I write this, no suspects for this killing have been arrested. Still, I had my own reward: the contentment of having done the best I could, of making the evidence reveal its secrets so that justice—whatever it was—could be done. I can't reveal any more about this open case, but suffice it to say that there is no statute of limitations on murder, and tomorrow always brings another day and another chance.

•   •   •

Tomorrow also seems always to bring another case. In my first six months on the job, I had to deal with the exhumation of an allegedly battered child who had been buried in 1972; a partially skeletonized victim tied to a tree and shot in the head; a corpse hidden in a refrigerator for a year; a decomposed body found in the Cumberland River; one case of skeletal remains slashed by a farm implement; another battered and left along the side of the road; and a third left scattered in the woods. Before the end of 1994, I also had to deal with eight separate cases in which fire had reduced the bodies to bone. Seven of these were probably tragic accidents, but one was definitely a homicide disguised by fire. Three mountain men blown to bits by land mines in a booby-trapped marijuana patch rounded out the census for that first half year.

With this kind of caseload, it didn't take me long to understand why Kentucky needed a full-time forensic anthropologist. Kentucky has a history of violent crime and "mountain justice" dating back even before the notorious feuds of the Hatfields and the McCoys. This culture of lawlessness has only gotten worse with the rise of illegal drug use and marijuana's dubious honor as the one of the Commonwealth's most lucrative cash crops. Add to that the region's large areas with limited access—perfect for hiding dead bodies—and a warm climate that needs only days to reduce a body to bones, and you have the ideal conditions to produce lots and lots of skeletal remains.

Sometimes the bones I look at are not recent victims but rather are ancient or historic bones that turn up during construction projects or archaeological digs. I try to refer those cases to one of Kentucky's many expert archaeologists or physical anthropologists, people whose academic training suits them to that type of analysis. I stick to bones that tell the stories of more recent crimes, though I occasionally consult with the academics to take advantage of their expertise.

One such expert is Nancy Ross-Stallings, a bespectacled self-avowed science nerd who works out of the tiny community of Harrodsburg as a contract archaeologist. She first came to my aid in the winter of 1995, after I had spent two days in the woods of McCreary County, down in the Daniel Boone National Forest near the Tennessee line.

Bill Conley (not his real name) had disappeared in the summer of 1994. About six months later, his boyfriend admitted to Lexington police detectives that he had killed Bill and hidden his body in the woods near Whitley City, another small town in southeastern Kentucky. State police troopers, sheriff's deputies, and Lexington city detectives searched diligently for Conley for more than a year, until finally, late one December afternoon in 1995, I got a call from the McCreary County Sheriff's Department. Conley's body was long gone, of course. But they thought they'd found his skull.

It was just before dark that I met Deputy David Morrow at the Blue Heron Café on Highway 27S. I followed his cruiser up a winding gravel road, where we stopped beside a pea-green 4x4 Jeep Cherokee belonging to the U.S. Forest Service. Through bitter experience, I'd learned to keep all of my key field gear in a sturdy backpack—in Kentucky's rough rural terrain, it's a rare occasion when I can actually drive my full-size van right up to a crime scene—so it didn't take long to transfer my camera, pack, and shovel into the Jeep.

A few minutes later, we had driven up the rocky, washed-out side road to a place where two trees had been marked with fluorescent orange spray paint, showing where one of the deputies had already blazed a path to the scene. I'd earned the nickname "Boondock Bone Doc" from all the hours I'd logged at crime scenes just like this one, on the side of a mountain or way out in the woods, searching for skeletal remains. And no matter where I went, no matter how isolated the scene, the first thing I always saw was a cluster of cops standing around smoking cigarettes, waiting patiently for my arrival.

"I hope this really is Conley's skull," I said under my breath to the deputy, and he nodded. During the past year, people searching for this very victim had located the skeletal remains of three *other* people in the woods within a thirty-mile radius of where we were right now. I couldn't help being a little skeptical.

"So how do you know it's his?" I went on.

David was just now getting his long legs untangled from the Jeep's backseat. He handed me my pack and smiled. "You see that scraggly lookin' guy by that tree?"

I nodded.

"He's says he's the one who killed him."

"You're kidding!"

"Yeah, he's been telling every cop who would listen that he killed his lover in Lexington, then brought the body down here to hide it. Unfortunately, he hid it so well that even *he* couldn't find it again, even after he decided to confess."

"Why did he confess?" I asked. "If the victim was so well hidden, no one would ever have been the wiser."

David laughed and leaned down to whisper in my ear. "The guy has AIDS now, and I guess he figured if he could get arrested and put in jail, then at least he'd have medical care for the rest of his life."

"Oh, great. And here I thought maybe he just felt guilty and wanted to do the right thing."

"Well, he did do the right thing, for whatever reason. We just need the body before we can put him away. Luckily, the detective in Lexington finally had him talk to one of the Forest Service guys who knows this area, and the killer's description of the terrain gave him just enough clues that he was able to find this skull. There's a side story to this too, that will make your hair stand on end—"

McCreary County Coroner Milford Creekmore joined us, interrupting the "side story" as he and his team piled out of their ancient ambulance, deluging us with friendly greetings. I stared at his old vehicle, hardly able to believe he'd gotten up into this rough terrain, but I should have known that where Milford was concerned, ordinary rules don't apply. We'd already worked together on a few cases—he's a great guy and, until his defeat in a close election a few years ago, he was one of Kentucky's most colorful coroners. Mountain born and bred, Milford was about as round as he was tall, and by age forty he'd lost all but a few of his natural teeth. He scrounged the junkyard for cheap vehicles and then equipped them with the most outlandish, jury-rigged set of lights and sirens you could imagine. However, tonight he had managed to get his vehicle up that terrible road, urging it on like a recalcitrant mule, and when he and his clan piled out I knew that not one of them would hang back from the work ahead, not Milford—or his two sons—or his ex-wife—or his daughter, who had brought along her baby. They all wanted to see the skull and help with the investigation, but Milford made it clear that he and no one else was going to be my right-hand man.

Walking single file through a steady cold drizzle, we all headed for the site, which was about twenty feet down the side of the embankment away from the road. A bright-orange surveyor's plastic flag marked the spot, and I was surprised that I couldn't see the skull—until Gus Skinner, the Forest Service law enforcement investigator, got down on his knees and folded back some droopy clumps of grass to reveal something resembling a groundhog's burrow. There, about two feet below the surface, I could see the back of a human skull, resting face down in a pool of crystal-clear water.

To reach into the hole—the origin of a little artesian spring—I'd have to lie down flat on my belly and stick one arm and shoulder into the burrow, with my cheek rubbing into the very soil where the victim's body had probably decomposed. Maybe I was getting used to human decay—but I wasn't yet ready to do *that*.

As soon as he saw the problem, Milford voluntarily removed his ample raincoat and laid it on the ground with a flourish that would have made Sir Walter Raleigh proud. I lay down on it, took a few pictures, and finally reached down to grab the skull. I sat up as quickly as I could, turning the skull over in my hands to do a brief analysis in the flashing light of the detectives' cameras.

First off, I could tell this skull had belonged to an adult White male—the same biological profile as the putative victim. I could see the empty tooth sockets with their sharply defined edges—clear signs that the man's teeth had fallen out after he died. I suspected that the teeth were still down there in the hole. I could also see one tooth socket that was already filling in with bone as the edges began to smooth over. *That* tooth had been lost well before death, so long ago, in fact, that it had begun to heal. The dental information would come in handy when we had to make our ID.

I didn't see any fresh fractures in the skull that would have indicated any sort of head injuries. That, too, was useful, because it told us that we wouldn't have to look for a bullet or a baseball bat.

I put the skull into my evidence bag for future reference and turned my attention to the teeth and some small neck bones I could now see at the bottom of the spring. Even when I lay on Milford's raincoat, they remained just out of my reach. The guys dug out a little around the hole's edge, which seemed like a good idea until I actually put my head, shoulders, and both arms into the enlarged hole. Then, thanks to Milford's plastic coat, I started to slide in, headfirst. Chivalry is not dead in Kentucky, though, and at least three pairs of hands instantly grabbed hold of my belt, ankles, and parts in between, saving me from a chilly, stinky shampoo.

With that we decided to quit for the night and start fresh the next morning. Milford made arrangements for all of us to stay at a little local motel and, after we checked in, we all slipped over to the café next door. By "all," I include the confessed murderer. In fact, sitting across from him, munching on my hamburger and talking about the weather, I lost sight of the fact that I was in the middle of a homicide investigation until he stood up, ostensibly to go to the bathroom. Three men with guns and badges were on their feet before he ever cleared his chair. He wasn't fazed by this, but I certainly was. When they finally escorted him to the men's room, the rest of us laughed quietly to break the tension. Then Deputy David Morrow leaned across the table and asked me if I wanted to hear the story he'd started to tell me out there in the woods. Of course, I said yes.

"I'm not sure you noticed, but halfway down that mountain road there was a divot in the limestone cliff, and a piece of pipe was sticking out," he began.

"Yeah, I saw that. It looked like some sort of well, or maybe a spring."

"That's exactly what it is, Doc, the outlet of a spring where most of the locals get their drinking water." In the next seat, Skinner, the weather-worn U.S. Forest Service investigator, nodded as he, too, listened intently.

"That spring is a dandy, too," chimed in Milford's son Ethelbert. "In fact, I stopped on my way down and filled me up a couple of jugs."

The deputy and Skinner exchanged glances. David set down his cup of coffee and closed his eyes. Skinner took over.

"Son, do you remember last spring when I placed a Forest Service warning sign on that spring?"

"Sure do. And do you know, the whole county was laughing at you for doing it? We've been getting our water from that spring ever since Daddy's daddy can remember. Everybody knows that it tastes funny every once in a while when the weather changes, but no harm has ever come of it. No gov'ment sign can keep the folks from this county from doin' what they've always done. And that's why that sign saying the water ain't fit to drink came down almost as soon as it went up."

"Well, Ethelbert, they shouldn't have done that," Skinner said patiently. "And you might want to go empty your jugs. Tonight the doc there almost fell into the source of that spring. And the guy she was trying to lift out of the water had a full-blown case of AIDS when the killer dumped his body there."

Everybody at the table froze, and we "outsiders" turned to look at the Creekmores sitting at one end of the long table. As one, they pushed back their chairs and left the café. It's hard to say what happened that night, but rumor has it that the phone lines in McCreary County were jammed for hours.

The next morning, though, they were all back at the site, ready to go to work. Nobody mentioned the fouled drinking water again, but when Milford, Jr., one of the hardest workers in the bunch, was helping me scour the sand and gravel from the little stream, a frown was fixed across his face and he never uttered a word.

We searched for bones until the middle of the afternoon and we were able to find about half of what Conley had started with. The forest carnivores—coyotes, foxes, raccoons, and opossums—had done their best to scatter individual bones as they dragged them away from the rotting carcass to feast on the flesh and gnaw for the marrow. Then Mother Nature camouflaged what was left. Leaf-fall had blanketed the forest floor, and the bones had bleached and discolored until they matched the deep gray-brown of the twigs and leaves that covered them.

Those bones' size and shape make some of them difficult to locate, and even when they *are* located, it's important not to pick them up right away. Earlier, I had handed out handfuls of brightly colored surveyor's flags to all of my helpers, instructing them to leave each bone where they found it. "Just stick a flag in the ground and call me," I'd urged. Sometimes, if you stand back and see the location of several bones at once, you can establish a pattern to the scatter. In many cases, heavy rains rushing down a slope or an animal following some instinctive route will scatter the bones in a specific direction that might lead you to a cache of smaller, lighter bones, the ones that are usually hardest to find.

That's exactly what had happened here, and after about fifteen flags dotted the forest floor, I could see that they formed a kind of pie-slice shape, with the apex right near the spot where we'd found the skull. From there, the flags sort of fanned out, with one edge of the triangle along the creek and the other at the base of the hill. We'd found one rib bone about sixty feet from the spring outlet, which we used to mark the third side of the triangle. For now, this triangle was the outer limit of our search as we walked shoulder to shoulder in one long line, back and forth across this wedge of land, stirring the leaves with our feet and sticking marker flags into the ground every time we found a bone.

The detectives took lots of pictures and then sketched the overall scene to document the bones' distribution. When we were finally ready to collect the bones, Milford, David, and I walked through the woods together. I picked up each bone, looked at it quickly, and told David how to enter it in the log book: #1 = right scapula, #2 = left humerus, and so on. Milford then popped each bone into a bag numbered according to the log.

Things had been going smoothly when I picked up #63, a left femur. When I looked at it, however, I was startled. What in the world had happened to the distal end of this bone, down by the knee? It looked as though it had been broken off, crisscrossed with deep gashes that left long bony splinters hanging off the end where the knee joint should have been. I knew these woods were full of black bears and coydogs—large mongrel farm dogs that had bred with coyotes—and I knew that these scavengers often chewed human bones down to the core. But this bone looked as though something else had happened to it.

I didn't want to slow down our search, so I just asked David to make a note in the log and told Milford to set this bone aside for a closer look. Then, about ten feet farther on, I picked up the right femur and the mystery began to clear up. This bone had identical striations and the end with the knee joint was also missing. I decided not to voice the suspicion that was beginning to form—not until we collected the rest of the evidence.

By now, the afternoon was turning to evening, and we had reached the point of diminishing returns. The rest of the team had searched an area about fifty yards beyond our triangle, and a local search and rescue team had brought in some of their cadaver dogs. All of these searchers now agreed that they'd done all they could and we decided to call it quits. We had enough bones and teeth to identify the victim, and we'd certainly recovered a great deal of Conley's skeleton.

I was no longer surprised, though, that we hadn't recovered any bones from Conley's feet or lower legs. Sitting down in the open rear hatch of the Jeep, I pulled out the two femurs, gently brushed off the dirt and leaf litter, and held them side by side. I could now be sure that the gashes and grooves were deliberate and man-made. Conley's legs had been cut off.

This was my first case of human butchering, and when I gathered my colleagues to explain my findings, they were as shocked and confused as I was. Of course, the murderer had already confessed, but none of us was comfortable with the notion that there was another crime scene out there somewhere—the place where someone had cut Conley's legs off at or around the time of death.

The Lexington detectives had already returned to their home turf, taking the confessed killer with them. David got through to them on his radio to see if they could squeeze any more information from the suspect before he "lawyered up." But our luck had run out. The confessed killer wasn't talking anymore, now that he was assured a lifelong berth in the penitentiary, and we were left to wonder what had happened. Maybe the body wouldn't fit into the trunk of his car once rigor mortis set in? Maybe he'd wanted to keep a trophy? Maybe he'd gotten hungry and decided to follow in the footsteps of Jeffrey Dahmer?

It's a safe bet that no one will ever know, but here's where I decided to call on Nancy, who I thought could at least help me identify the weapon that had been used to make the cuts. Nancy had studied the macabre practice of human butchering and the evidence this practice left on bones—just the kind of science that I needed to wrap up this case.

When Nancy had a chance to examine the bones, she confirmed that the preliminary cuts on Bill's legs had been made with a thick, smooth-bladed knife, while the final amputations had been performed with hacking blows from an axe-like tool. She explained that a saw or a knife often leaves its "signature" on the bone, so that a hacksaw, for instance, makes fine irregular lines across the cut end of a bone, whereas a large table saw cuts cleanly in a single direction until the bone is severed. A chainsaw rips and chews through the bone in an instant, leaving gouges and chips in its wake, while a serrated knife leaves a pattern of dips and points—not to be confused with the straight, smooth cut mark often left by a butcher knife or a meat cleaver. The work done with cut marks by Nancy and my fellow forensic anthropologists—Steve Symes of Pennsylvania and the late William Maples of Florida—has helped to put numerous suspects behind bars.

I've had occasion to use cut-mark evidence in several other Kentucky cases, in sometimes surprising ways. One of the things that haunts investigators is knowing that a person can die violently—stabbed, shot, poisoned—without a single mark being left on the bone. And when the flesh has decomposed or been burned away, the bones are all you've got left.

Luckily, bones enable you to roughly determine the time a wound was inflicted, and fairly easily, too, because the nature of bone changes so radically after the body dies. When a person is alive or very recently dead, his or her bones resemble green wood. If you stick a knife into what we call a "green bone," you can pry up a little sliver, because the bone—living tissue—is still pliable. If you try to make the same cut days or weeks after death, the bone is more like firewood—dead and dried-out wood—and it's not going to have that flexibility. That's why the cut marks made at or around the time of death look completely different from those made after death—if you know what to look for. So when Nancy and I reviewed the evidence in the case of Bill Conley, we concluded that the bone had been sliced "perimortem"—either at the time of death, immediately before, or fairly soon thereafter.

Although we couldn't tell exactly why the amputation had happened, at least Nancy had identified the butchering tools.

•   •   •

From a death investigator's point of view, there are two types of fires: the kind that kill people, and the kind that somebody sets to disguise a homicide. Kentucky has far more than its share of the latter, and nobody really knows why. Is it that investigators in other states just aren't as suspicious about fire-related deaths as we are? Or does the criminal element in Kentucky really not know that even the most all-consuming fire inevitably leaves behind some human bones?

Of course, I'm glad they don't know. I'm kind of reluctant to tell them. But for the record, here it is: If you ever plan to incinerate a person, don't count on the body being completely destroyed. Trying to burn a human body—which after all is about 80 percent water—is like trying to burn a huge, sopping sponge. The fluid-filled organs, muscles, and bones can often withstand the fiercest of flames.

Ironically, one of my first major cases of homicide disguised by fire also happened in Pulaski County, where it was initially discovered by my old friend Sheriff Sam Catron. By the time this case broke in 1995, Sam, like so many law enforcement officers in Kentucky, had learned to keep my personal phone numbers in his pocket. My colleagues across the state know I'm available to them at any time of the day or night, so I wasn't surprised to get Sam's call at five o'clock one April Sunday afternoon.

"So here's the story," Sam said wearily after we'd exchanged the usual pleasantries. "A small wood-frame farmhouse in the northeastern corner of the county burned to the ground earlier this afternoon. The fire department found two charred bodies in the living room. We found one more in one of the bedrooms."

Sam and I both knew that this case wasn't necessarily a homicide. In Kentucky, it's not that unusual for remote dwellings to burn to the ground with sleeping or incapacitated occupants inside. Lots of mountain folks rely on wood-burning stoves and kerosene heaters for heat, and they sometimes use coal-oil lamps or even candles for light. The rural volunteer fire departments do their best, but sometimes they're not even aware of the fire until it's too late to help. In this case, a distant neighbor just happened to see the blaze and call it in. But the ramshackle old house was pretty much rubble by the time the firefighters got there.

Generally, the coroner, local law enforcement officers, and an arson specialist examine a fire scene. If the fire appears to be truly accidental, the bodies are simply recovered and brought to the M.E.'s office for autopsy and positive ID.

So what had made Sam and the coroner suspicious in this case? For one thing, the fire had occurred in the middle of a mild day in April. Not much chance that anyone was using a heater. Then there was the time of day. How likely was it that three able-bodied people were sleeping so soundly during daylight hours that they couldn't make their way out of this small one-story house, especially since there were plenty of doors and windows? The third clue, and the one most significant to trained fire-death investigators, was the fact that the bodies themselves were in abnormal positions.

Of course, probably no charred fire victim can be said to have a "normal" position, but there are certain things you look for when investigating a fire death. If a person dies from smoke inhalation—the usual cause of death in a fire—carbon monoxide builds up in the blood, causing a rapid loss of consciousness. Even after the person has blacked out, though, his or her body continues to react. The windpipe, or trachea, sucks in soot and smoke, and the organs and muscles turn a bright cherry red as carbon monoxide replaces oxygen in the blood. Last-minute chemical reactions in the muscles of the victim cause him or her to contort into what we call the "pugilistic" position—arms bent at the elbows; wrists and forearms drawn in toward the shoulders; hands balled into fists, as if the person were engaged in a boxing match. The legs, too, often flex slightly at the hips and the knees, so that the victim looks to be sitting in some imaginary chair.

However, none of the bodies in the Pulaski County farmhouse were in that position, Sam told me, meaning that there had been no physiological muscle reactions to the fire. And since Sam could actually see one victim's internal organs through rents in the abdominal wall, he'd noticed that there was no sign of the cherry-red discoloration that would have been there if the victim had died while inhaling smoke.

When I arrived at the scene, Sam walked me through the remnants of the little house and pointed out the other reasons he was suspicious. Something about this case had gotten to him: There was a catch in his normally soft voice, lending an air of uncharacteristic sadness to a man I had come to know as cheerful and completely professional even at a crime scene. Then, as we tiptoed through the rubble, Sam suddenly bent down beside a bright-yellow marker flag, and I saw what had affected this career lawman so profoundly. This victim was tiny—by my estimation, a child no older than two or three.

"There's another little one over here, Doc," Sam said as he took my hand and helped me negotiate over a still-smoking pile of rubble topped off with a porcelain sink. This second victim was a little bigger, but from head to toe, he—or she—was only about four feet long.

"I know you don't like us to go tromping around through a fire when we've got potential murder victims," Sam went on. "So once the coroner and I confirmed that we had a suspicious situation, I had everybody just back off until you got here. But the biggest body is over there." He pointed with his chin while lifting a burned beam out of our way. "Firefighters found that one right off—the others were so little that it took a while. But nothing's been disturbed. Even the firefighters stopped spraying heavy water once they realized there were bodies in here, just a fine mist to keep the fire down."

Sam stopped talking abruptly as though he was trying to get control of his voice, and I had to stifle an impulse to put a comforting hand on his arm. Instead, keeping my own voice casual, I said, "Okay, Sam, that's good. Why don't you keep filling me in while I'm getting my stuff together?"

Sam followed me out to my van, talking more naturally now. "The neighbor says that a woman, Shirley Bowles, lived here with her two kids, Amy and Brian. Seems she got married to man she hardly knew back about a month ago, 'cause she thought he could help her out with the kids. That man, McKinney, was around when they were trying to put out the fire, but he left when the firemen started asking the whereabouts of Shirley and the little ones. He came back for a while, but then when they started finding bodies, he disappeared for good."

I cast a furtive glance into the woods, which were turning dark with the setting sun. "Where is he now?"

Sam saw what I was thinking and, suddenly, he grinned. "I don't know, Doc, but I've got men out looking for him. I've also got sharpshooters posted around this place, just in case he tries something funny. You know I always cover your back."

He was right there. Once, his deputies had literally shielded my body with their own when a distraught father had sneaked up to the periphery of our crime scene with a rifle, threatening to shoot me and the coroner during our court-ordered exhumation of his two children.

I grinned back. "Okay, Sam. How about you watch out for me, and I'll try to help us nail whoever did this?"

I climbed into the one-piece navy jumpsuit I wear at most crime scenes, along with the matching cap that proudly announced "State Medical Examiner." After I pulled on my fireproof boots, I strapped heavy pads across the front of my knees so I could crawl over anything in my path, pulled on a pair of thin leather gloves, and reached for a stack of the plastic snap-lid boxes I keep in my van for collecting fire-scene evidence.

Back in the house, I knelt beside the biggest victim and lifted off the large pieces of burned wood that had half-buried the body. Then I gently brushed away the loose debris from what used to be the victim's face with a large, soft paintbrush about four inches wide, careful not to disturb any bone fragments that might be in the vicinity. Like any housewife, I brushed the ashes into an ordinary dustpan, and then— contrary to most standard housekeeping manuals—slid them carefully into a paper bag to look at later under a magnifying lens.

The victim's face had all burned away, but I could see by her bones that she was a female. What remained of her forehead was smooth and rounded, or "bossed," while the bone above her eye sockets was smooth, without the heavy brow ridge that most men have. Her bones also told me that she was an adult: Her skull bones and their connecting growth plates, or suture lines, showed signs of complete closure, as opposed to a child's partially open skull. And this woman's mouth was clearly full of permanent teeth. A large section of her skull was missing, but I could see the broken fragments—some still attached to her body, others scattered among the debris. Rearing back on my haunches, I tried to keep my hands and body out of the way as I asked the detective standing beside me to take several photos.

When I'm working a crime scene—especially a fire scene, where all the evidence is so fragile—I continually have to remind myself and everyone else to *slow down*. After all, the victims are already dead. They're not going to get any deader. Despite the natural human reaction to respect the dead by removing and cleaning up their bodies as soon as possible, we actually show them more respect by leaving them where they are and documenting the evidence that can help us discover how they died. Once you've moved a piece of evidence at a crime scene, that's it. You can never put it back.

To make sure we all take proper care, I've developed my own protocol for collecting evidence from a suspicious fire-death scene, a procedure that has proven to be so successful that coroners across the Commonwealth have adopted it as the standard for all fire deaths. Better safe than sorry and, if an apparent accident turns out to be murder, this procedure will protect what might turn out to be crucial evidence.

So now, having exposed the body and noted its position and condition, I continued to follow my own protocol. First stop: the head, where I tried to pick up fragments that might have separated from the rest of the skull. Several of these quarter-sized broken pieces had already fallen into the pile of burned debris that surrounded the victim's head and shoulders. Other pieces teetered precariously on the rounded surface of the remaining skull, so before they could fall, I gen-

tly coaxed them free and stored them in one of the snap-lid boxes that
were also part of my protocol. Before I started using these boxes, fragments were simply placed in the body bag, where they were often
ground into powder from their contact with other bones and the body
itself during the long, bumpy journey from the crime scene to the
morgue. I quickly learned not to do that, because I know these loose
fragments are too precious to lose: By putting them back together at
the autopsy, I often figure out exactly how the person died. The boxes
are a great protector, and I'm happy their use has spread across the
state.

Meanwhile, the woman's partially destroyed head lay before me, so
I picked up a small piece of skull bone from the ashes and matched its
jagged edges to the part of the skull still clinging to her brain. These
two bone fragments had once formed a single bone—but the piece I
held in my hand was a pale, toasty brown, while the piece attached to
her brain was charred and blackened by the fire. The bone had been
cleanly fractured and was easy to rematch—but why were the two fragments such different colors? The answer to that question lay in the science of differential burning.

Differential burning is most often associated with fatal wounds to the
skull, that prime target of murderers. Usually, when you're dealing
with a fire, you're trying to answer one key question: Did the intense
heat of the fire break this skull apart, or was the skull shot, hit, or
crushed *before* the fire began?

If you know how to read the skull fragments, they can usually tell
you. When an intact skull cracks open in a fire, all the pieces show the
same kind of burning, as if a painted vase had simply cracked. If the
skull was fractured before it burned, however, each fragment burns in
a slightly different way. When you reconstruct that kind of skull, it
looks as though somebody broke a vase, painted a few random pieces,
and then put it back together.

That sort of differential burning was here in my hands, and since we
all knew something wasn't quite right with this scene, I didn't want to
take any chances on losing what might be a crucial piece of evidence.

So I got Alan Stringer's brother, Larry, the deputy coroner, to help me with the next step. Larry gently lifted the victim's rigid shoulders, bringing the head up out of the burned debris as I unfolded a medium-sized white trash bag, the kind that has a built-in drawstring at one end, and slipped it over her head. Now if anything else broke off, it would be preserved intact inside the bag. And if any associated evidence should get dislodged during transport—a tooth, an earring, maybe even the bullet or bullet fragments I was seeking—that would be safely contained as well.

With the victim's head tightly wrapped in plastic, I picked up the pieces of bone at the distal, or far, ends of her arms and legs. This was harder than it sounds. Imagine a fireplace in which all the wood has burned away to ash and clinkers. Now you have to go through those clinkers—all of them the same color; each with its own odd, distorted shape—and distinguish between the ones that used to be bone and the ones that used to be wood. They all look pretty much the same, so your only clue is a variation in shape—and, of course, each piece's relationship to the torso.

Working as slowly and carefully as I could and documenting each part of the process, I recovered the bones of each extremity—left arm and hand, left leg and foot, then the right arm, the right leg, putting each extremity into its own carefully labeled plastic box. I took special care with the victim's right arm, where I could see some differences in color in the bone fragments, which again suggested differential burning. My guess was that her arm, too, had been broken into pieces before it burned off in the fire.

With all the small pieces recovered, we were finally ready to bag the torso. I'd learned the hard way to save that for last, having seen many cases in which grabbing the torso first disrupted forever the fragile, fire-ravaged bones of the extremities.

Now the body was gone—but we still weren't through with this victim's associated evidence. Because of the numerous fractures, I strongly suspected that this woman had sustained at least one gunshot wound to the head and one to the arm, so we scooped up the charred and blackened debris that had lain under the victim, hoping it contained a bullet.

Whenever a person is shot, you hope that the bullet is still inside the body. When the body is burned, though, a bullet might fall through the charred flesh into the surrounding debris. I can't stand the thought of losing a bullet, so when I work a potential homicide scene, I make sure to shovel up all of the debris, load it into bags, boxes, or buckets, and take it back with me to the lab. There an x-ray will point me to any bullets or parts thereof. In this case, we'd bagged up the body and the debris—but what if a bullet had passed all the way through the body and landed elsewhere in the mess? Sam and I were taking no chances: The house would remain a protected crime scene until after the autopsies. If I had to come back and put every scrap of wood and ash through a fine archaeological sifter, I was fully prepared to do so.

By the time I finished the recovery and field analysis of the children, I could see they'd most likely suffered the same fate as their mother. As I shared my suspicions with the rest of the team, our determination grew. We were all more than willing to do whatever it took to make sure someone didn't get away with murder. Not this time.

By now, I'd been on the job long enough to realize that most investigators—myself included—tend to divide cases into two categories. There are the ordinary murders, the ones you want to solve but have to accept that you might not. And—even though you always remain impartial with the evidence—there are some cases that really get to you, the ones you know will trouble your sleep for months to come if you don't put the killer behind bars. This was one of those cases. A young woman and two innocent children had apparently been gunned down and then incinerated—and not one seasoned professional at that scene was going to rest until we'd found out who'd done it.

It was after midnight when I got home that night, and the odor of burned flesh, smoke, and blood had seeped into my nose, my skin, and even my hair. I showered for at least thirty minutes, trying to remove the scent of death, until I finally realized the taint was no longer on my body but had burned into my brain. Those weeks in Texas, the bodies of burned children, the odors of singed hair and charred flesh, engulfed me in a flashback that I couldn't repress. I crawled into bed and cried myself to sleep—something I hadn't done since Waco. Luckily, sleep worked its healing magic and I awoke the next morning ready to face a new day.

.   .   .

Less than a week later, Gary Casper McKinney, husband and stepfather of the victims, was arrested, and in 1998 he was on trial, facing three charges of capital murder and multiple other charges, including tampering with physical evidence, arson, and abuse of a corpse. The courtroom testimony mesmerized Pulaski County for more than a week, drawing spectators who filled the churchlike pews, curious to hear what had really happened there on Poplar Bluff Road on that quiet Sunday afternoon. The crowd was divided, somewhat like a rural wedding service, with friends and family of the victims on one side of the room and McKinney's kin on the other.

The sheriff, his deputies, and the arson and ballistics experts testified one by one. Then it was my turn. We each presented evidence that was pertinent to the case, even playing a videotape of the crime scene that showed men removing the charred bodies from the burned-out structure. When Drs. Hunsaker and Coyne, the two forensic pathologists, gave their testimony, the defendant's fate was sealed. The vivid description of mother Shirley Bowles's death from multiple gunshot wounds was gripping enough, but no one even seemed to breathe as Dr. John Hunsaker revealed that a gun had pumped three bullets directly into the top of eleven-year-old Brian's head. Moments later a gasp echoed throughout the courtroom when Dr. Carolyn Coyne revealed that three-year-old Amy had died instantly after the trigger was pulled on a gun that had been thrust into her mouth.

The day I testified, Sam was waiting for me outside the courtroom.

He came up to me, extending his right hand for a handshake and putting his other hand on my shoulder. We stood there looking at each other for the longest time, and I could see the tears in his eyes. "Thanks, Doc," he said finally, and squeezed my hand one last time before he walked away.

After eight days of testimony and only five hours of deliberation, the jury found McKinney guilty of all three murders and he was sentenced to death. It was the first triple death sentence that anyone could remember in the history of the Pulaski County Circuit Court.

· · ·

The Pulaski murder was the last one I ever cried over—until my friend Sam himself was assassinated in April 2002. Sam's life was ended abruptly by a sniper's bullet as he was leaving a rally and fish fry held during his campaign for a fifth term as sheriff.

Kenneth White, one of the biggest drug dealers and bootleggers in the county, thought that if Sam was out of the way, a more pliable sheriff might be elected, someone who would look the other way at the criminal activity in Pulaski County. White managed to get one of his henchmen, a former sheriff's deputy, named Jeff Morris, on the ballot, but it soon became clear that no one could beat Sam Catron in a fair election. So White and Morris decided to take more desperate measures. Danny Shelley, a local addict, seemed to be the perfect pawn in their plan, so they convinced him that Sam would kill him if he didn't kill Sam first. On that fateful night, Shelley pulled the trigger from a wooded hilltop overlooking the site of the fish fry and then sped off on White's motorcycle. Men in pickup trucks took off after him, and after a high-speed chase through the mountains, Shelley crashed. The impromptu posse pinned him down until he could be handcuffed and arrested by Sam's deputies.

Shelley almost immediately told authorities all about the scheme, then pled guilty before his case could go to trial. Eventually Morris also pled guilty, but White decided to take his chances before a jury. After more than a week of testimony, that jury took less than an hour to convict and sentence White to life in prison with no possibility of parole.

Sam was a beloved figure throughout the state and was nationally known for his dedication, honesty, and skill. The brutality—and the stupidity—of his assassination sent shock waves through the nation and the world, with his death receiving coverage from as far away as England, Poland, and Russia. More than two thousand mourners turned out for his funeral, and the Kentucky state legislature adjourned for a full day in his honor.

Whenever I think of Sam, I remember the day we were working a case we called "River Legs," after a pair of decomposed legs that some canoeist had found floating down the Rockcastle River. Sam, Coroner Alan Stringer, and I went down to the river with several deputies to look for the rest of the remains.

The Rockcastle was a real wilderness river, deep down in a ravine, with high banks on each side. Sam and Alan flew reconnaissance, looking for other body parts in Sam's Huey helicopter, a craft he'd learned to fly so he could patrol his large rural county for signs of marijuana growing. I was out on a huge rock at the river's edge, flat on my belly, peering into the clear water with my binoculars—when suddenly I looked up in alarm. Sam and Alan had been flying low, of course, but now they were *too* low, the helicopter flying straight at me at what seemed an incredible rate. I later learned that Alan, who'd never been in a helicopter before, had shifted his weight unthinkingly, resting his thigh on the helicopter's collective, which controls its flight. With Alan's weight on the collective, Sam couldn't pull out of the deadly trajectory—and from what I could see, the helicopter was going to kill me for sure. But they flew so close in their open craft that I could look right into Sam's eyes—and then I wasn't frightened anymore. I just knew by the flicker in his stare that Sam would put that helicopter in the river before he let it hit me. And at the *last* possible instant—I mean, that thing was blowing river water into my eyes—Sam reached over and somehow pulled Alan off the collective. The craft whizzed right on by me. I was all right.

"Sorry to scare you, Doc," Sam said when we all met up on solid ground later that day.

"I wasn't scared," I answered, and we both knew I was telling the truth.

•   •   •

Losing Sam has given me a little bit of insight into what the relatives of homicide victims go through. I wasn't sure I could make it through his funeral. I wouldn't have missed it, though—and I'm so glad I went. My law enforcement colleagues welcomed me like a sister, and I knew once and for all that I was finally part of their community. That, I guess, was Sam's last gift to me.

5

A Single Death

A single death is a tragedy, a million deaths is a statistic.
— JOSEPH STALIN

I'VE ALWAYS LIKED to work jigsaw puzzles. I like looking at the picture on the box and then trying to make hundreds of oddly shaped pieces add up to one coherent image. I enjoy that chaotic period at the beginning when all the little bits look alike and you have to keep a sharp eye out for the ones with straight edges that go around the border, or the light-blue ones that are probably the sky. And I get an enormous amount of satisfaction from putting in the final piece so that the picture is finally complete.

I've often thought that my work as a forensic anthropologist resembles a four-dimensional jigsaw puzzle. A series of events happened: Somewhere back in time someone was murdered or died violently, or maybe even died peacefully, leaving behind a few bones or some body

parts. Days, weeks, or even years later, I come along and try to reconstruct the picture on the box, using whatever pieces I can find: a bone,
a skull, a broken plant, a pile of ashes, perhaps a personal possession or
two. I'm looking at the evidence in front of me, and I'm also looking
back in time, trying to figure out how I can make the pieces fit, hoping that the picture I put together matches the events that really happened. When I start out, it's chaos. But when I finish, with any luck,
it all makes sense.

Of course, some cases are more like that than others. I think that the
most absorbing and intricate jigsaw puzzle I ever worked on was probably the case that began on April 21, 2000.

•   •   •

It started, as they all do, with a phone call. I carry a pager with me
twenty-four hours a day every single day of the year, and I never really
know what's in store for me when it goes off or when the phone rings.
It might be someone with a quick question, a detective calling about
some animal bones he just found. Or perhaps it's a complicated request
that I can nonetheless answer from the comfort of my home or office,
maybe from a coroner concerned about recovering victims' remains
after an accidental house fire. Sometimes I'll get an emergency call that
requires me to rush to a scene, a frantic 911 operator telling me that a
plane has just gone down in some remote rural area or a county official alerting me to incinerated occupants of a motor vehicle crash-and-
burn on the interstate. It can wreak havoc on my personal life. I've had
to cancel Saturday night dates, leave the grocery store with a half-filled
basket, and even pull a partly cooked roast out of the oven. If I'm in
Kentucky, I'm on call. The only respite I can count on is to leave the
Commonwealth for an occasional vacation, when I finally get to leave
my pager turned off for a while.

Usually, though, I'm ready and willing to respond to the crime
scene. My calls most often come from a coroner in one of Kentucky's
120 counties, asking me to come help out with a skeleton or decom-

posed human remains that have just been found in his or her jurisdiction. On this peaceful Saturday night, the call was from Campbell County Coroner Dr. Mark Schweitzer. Apparently two young boys fishing in the Ohio River late that afternoon had discovered the half-buried bones of a human skeleton.

By the time he called me, Mark had already been out to the site and confirmed that these were indeed human remains. He'd noticed, too, that the bones still seemed to be wearing some pants and a long-sleeved shirt.

"The clothing was a faded workman's blue," Mark told me. "But nobody's been reported missing lately. That area is kind of a hobo jungle—food cans scattered all over the place, lots of cheap liquor bottles, some plastic bags and dirty blankets. So the police think the bones belonged to some derelict who simply washed up onto the bank of the river and decomposed there, maybe a few months ago."

The Fort Thomas Police Department was already on the scene, Mark went on, with Detective Mike Daly in charge. Daly was pretty new to this type of investigation, having just been promoted to detective about six months ago. This was his first case of skeletal remains, and he was eager to prove that he could resolve this matter quickly and definitively.

"So," Mark concluded, "Daly and I figured we'd just bring those bones right down to your office."

"Don't you dare!" I said as playfully as I could. "I hope you haven't forgotten what I taught you." I tried to keep my tone friendly and patient, though at my end of the phone line I was rolling my eyes in exasperation. What *is* it about bones that makes people want to pick them up? Coroners who would never dream of disturbing other types of evidence seem to think nothing of gathering skeletal evidence and blithely removing it from the scene. Even experienced police investigators who know perfectly well that *they* need to see the crime scene exactly as the criminal left it don't quite understand why I, too, have to view the evidence in context.

At least in Mark's case, I could refer back to the advanced forensic anthropology workshops I'd taught, courses that he and his deputy, Al Garnick, had taken as part of the Kentucky Department of Criminal Justice's extensive coroner training program. My main objective in that class is to instill one key slogan in the mind of every death investigator in the Commonwealth: When you see bone, *leave it alone.*

Still, it took several heated phone calls, with Mark and Daly passing the phone back and forth between them, before the two men reluctantly agreed to wait until I got to the scene the next morning.

"I'll get there by dawn," I promised. "But this one isn't an emergency. There's just no reason to start recovering those bones at night." I wondered how much of their urgency was due to simple inexperience, colored by countless TV images of nighttime crime scenes. An immediate response makes all kinds of sense when you're dealing with a recent murder and a fresh corpse. But these bones had been buried in the dirt and covered with rotting cloth, and from Mark's description they were perched precariously on the banks of the rain-swollen Ohio River. That was a risky place to be even during the day, let alone in the middle of the night.

By the time we'd made our arrangements, it was close to midnight. I couldn't help feeling a bit wistful; the next day was Easter Sunday, and I'd been planning to attend a sunrise service, followed by an afternoon potluck barbecue with some friends in Bourbon County. Of course, nobody in law enforcement can ever count on personal plans, but at least cops have shifts.

I lay down and tried to get a few hours of sleep, but the adrenaline that accompanies every case had kicked in and my mind was racing. Mark had told me that these bones had been found in a quiet, secluded place totally hidden from the public eye, so it wouldn't be hard for Daly to secure the scene with a twenty-four-hour guard, as was required whenever human remains are found. Guarding a scene isn't so bad when it's in town and you've got dozens of cops milling around you, but I felt sorry for the poor guy assigned to overnight duty on this case, stuck way out in the woods somewhere with nothing to do but stare at some bones. He probably felt more like a babysitter than a cop.

In his place, I'd be bored out of my mind, so I always make a point of getting to the scene as early as possible. There was nothing we could do, though, till the sun came up. I found myself running over a mental checklist of what I'd need the next day, even though I knew my crime scene van was already stocked and ready to go, as it always is. When you get as many last-minute calls as I do, you find a way to stay permanently packed.

I tried to turn my mind off but it was probably 2 a.m. before I actually got to sleep, only two hours before the alarm blasted through my bedroom. After three smacks to the snooze button and a long, warm shower I was on the road by 5:00, feeling a fresh wave of adrenaline kick in. No matter how many times I've been called out on a case (and by the time I worked this one, the number was up in the hundreds), I always feel the same rush of excitement, the same thrill of the chase. I know the cops I work with feel the same excitement, along with firefighters, paramedics, and other emergency workers. Each of us knows and mourns the human tragedy involved, but to be honest, we also enjoy the adrenaline rush we experience: heart beating faster and harder, palms starting to sweat, brain and muscles all keyed up from an extra share of blood. The day I stop feeling that thrill is the day I go back to drawing medical pictures for a living.

I'd arranged to meet Mark and Al at Mark's home in Fort Thomas, and when I pulled into Mark's driveway in the darkness, I could see that this same kind of high had hit them too. Both men were waiting for me in the yard, finishing their first cup of coffee, and anxious to get started.

Mark was a good-looking young man with a winning smile and a flair for fashion, so I had to stifle a smile when I saw what he was wearing today. Like me, he was clothed in a jumpsuit, a garment designed to handle the mud, blood, and unidentified substances that abound at most crime scenes. In sharp contrast to my faded navy uniform, however, Mark was dressed in one of the most remarkable outfits I'd ever seen. It was brand-new, for starters, with razor-sharp creases ironed into the sleeves and trousers, and every inch of the khaki shirt was covered with shiny new decals, flags, and insignia. It looked as though it hadn't even been washed yet.

"I thought you said this case was in a rough spot," I said, trying to be tactful.

Mark smiled sheepishly. "Well, it is," he said, "but I've never worked a skeletal case in the woods before, so my wife thought this would be a good time to break in my field gear." He was so young and eager, I felt as if I were taking my kid brother off to scout camp. On the other hand, Al, the retired cop, his face creased from years of smoking and bad coffee, was wearing faded jeans, an old wool shirt, and a leather jacket I just knew was left over from World War II.

By seven o'clock, we had all reached the river, parking our separate vehicles in the dirt alongside the isolated road. As I got out of my van, I shivered from the wave of heavy fog that swirled up through the trees to greet me. It was still too dark to see more than a few feet ahead of us, so we groped our way along the bank until we reached the barrier of yellow crime-scene tape. Off in the woods, I could see a half-dozen tiny spots of light moving our way. They were cigarettes, I realized, in the hands of cops who had already gathered at the site. They'd heard us stumbling through the woods and came over to meet us, each with a cup of coffee in one hand, a cigarette in the other. They were obviously expecting us because they handed each of us a fresh cup as well, and that was all it took to make us members of the team.

We stood around waiting for the fog to clear, introducing ourselves, then starting in on the jokes and stories that always seem to bond this sort of work crew. Just as the coffee ran out, the fog started to lift, and we all slipped under the yellow crime-scene tape and moved cautiously toward the river. The officer who had spent the night at the scene led us to a steep ledge and pointed out the bright orange marker flags that Daly had placed there the night before. I could see exposed parts of the skeleton still embedded in the earth, a few bones perched precariously on chunks of sand that looked ready to break off and slide into the river. A little farther up the bank, more bones lay amid pieces of fabric.

I took a few steps back from the ledge and shook my head. Thank heavens we'd waited until it got light! Even during the daytime, recovering those bones would be a delicate, dangerous job, as my colleagues and I struggled to keep our footing on a slick, muddy riverbank that dropped about six feet straight down to the rain-swollen Ohio River. By the end of the day I knew I'd be exhausted from hours of trying to keep my balance, a trowel clutched in one hand, a safety rope wrapped around the other.

I opened up my backpack and pulled out what has become my standard working gear: thin leather gloves with the fingertips cut off, a length of rope, my kneepads, and a firefighter's belt. A few feet away, the cops watched me curiously, while I did my best to act nonchalant. Since I'm often attached to a climbing rope, grasping after the bones and body parts strewn with depressing regularity over Kentucky's big, green mountains and deep, dramatic ravines, this is routine for me, but the men sometimes seem mystified when they see me in this get-up.

"Hey, Al, give me a hand with this belt, will you?" I was taking no chances with the slick and crumbling riverbank. I looped the heavy webbing around my ample rear, pulled it tight around my waist, and clipped it onto the thick rope. Al obligingly wrapped the other end of the rope twice around a tree before grasping the other end firmly in his big hand. I could probably have stood upright even without the rope, but the small degree of constant tension helped me keep my balance and gave me that extra bit of psychological security I needed. I just prayed Al would have the strength to haul me up the bank if the soil gave out from under me.

If this had been a routine murder, every officer present would have known how to document the evidence and secure the scene. For some reason, though, bones seem to turn it into a whole new situation, so these experienced law-enforcement professionals were all looking to me.

"Okay, guys," I said to the assembled team. "The first thing we need is a videographer. And a photographer." It would be heartbreaking to spend hours recovering and analyzing skeletal evidence only to have it thrown out of court because someone hadn't recorded where, when, and how it was found.

Of course, the pictures, even those taken first thing this morning, would not show a pristine crime scene. There were footprints everywhere from all the people who'd been traipsing through the scene the previous evening. I didn't so much mind the folks who had legitimate tasks to perform, but I knew some of the prints had been left by cops who were just plain curious. I could read last night's frantic activity in the recently broken branches and plant stems throughout the area, and in the newly disturbed soil around the victim's skull.

At least the officers had established a definite perimeter, looping bright yellow tape around several trees and then stretching it taut to set off an area approximately of about 1,600 square feet. Any member of the public who showed up in this isolated spot would hopefully have been deterred by the large black letters warning CRIME SCENE—DO NOT CROSS.

Down by the river, most of the remains appeared to be untouched. Even from this distance, I could make out the soft mix of sand and mud that typifies the banks along the flood-prone Ohio River, and it was this fine-grained fluvial mix, soaked by recent rains, that made the riverbank so treacherous. In the places where the bank dropped steeply down to the river, the soft soil tended to break off under even the slightest pressure.

"Once I'm down there," I went on, "I'll have a better idea of what comes next." Grabbing a handful of marker flags, I let Al ease me down about twenty feet to the edge of the dropoff, where the bones were down a steady, steep slope, with an overhanging ledge that jutted out over a straight drop down to the river.

"All right," I called back up from the brink. "We don't really know what we've got yet, so we're going to have to document this just as if it's a homicide. I don't want it to get too crowded down here, so let's restrict access to the men taking the pictures. Oh, and let's have somebody taking notes and bagging the evidence. I'll recover the bones myself and hand them up to Mark." I took another look at the slick bank. "Somebody probably should be safety officer, too, just to keep an eye on things."

The officers looked at one another for a moment, then quickly divided up the tasks. Officer David Lambers of the Fort Thomas Police Department, a young, clean-cut kid with a shy, friendly demeanor, got the job of note-taker. He would also pack each bone into its own little evidence bag, labeling it carefully with the case number, time, and date. Two other officers picked up the cameras, while the remaining men formed a kind of bucket brigade, ready to pass each bone up the riverbank to the coroner.

As the guys quickly sorted themselves out, I was struck again by the difference between real life and TV, where you often see one single heroic scientist doing *all* the jobs at a crime scene, or micromanaging the cops with detailed orders. I don't do that. I concentrate on the evidence associated with the remains and try to capitalize on everyone else's special areas of expertise. I have an enormous amount of respect for the police, who know far better than I do how to document and process a crime scene. No fixed protocol works every time; each situation is unique, but you always need to remember, every step of the way, to keep a record of everything you do and of how things looked before you did it. As I recovered the bones, for example, I'd leave marker flags to show where the skull had been and how the bones had been scattered. After I collected the evidence, we'd take pictures of the flags and measure how far apart they were. If I ever had to testify in court where I found the skull, I wanted to be able to say something more precise than, "Um, I think it was kinda near the riverbank." "Seventy-two inches from Tree A, as labeled in this photograph taken on the morning of April 22," would make much better testimony.

The other golden rule of crime scenes is so obvious you'd think it wouldn't need to be mentioned: *Don't damage the evidence.* Yet detectives who understand this very well when the evidence is a drinking glass or a piece of jewelry tend to underestimate how fragile skeletal evidence can be. I didn't want one single mark on those bones that could be attributed either to me or my colleagues, and I was prepared to spend as long as I needed in the recovery process to guarantee that didn't happen.

•   •   •

Recovering human remains is always a fascinating experience, and new theories about the case can evolve as you come across new bits of evidence. That's how it was this day. When we started, we were looking at the fairly routine excavation of what was probably a derelict who had died peacefully (if tragically) within the past few months. By the end of the day, a series of small, odd, and fascinating clues had led us to suspect that this was one of the most unusual cases that any of us had ever worked on.

The skull was precariously close to the river's edge, so I decided to start with that. I was especially curious about a peculiar mass of whitish material that I could see on the ground around the skull. From a distance, it looked like adipocere, or grave wax, a grainy material that bears a weird resemblance to crumbling Styrofoam. You tend to find adipocere wherever body fat decomposes in a moist area containing abnormally low levels of oxygen, and I thought that its presence here helped confirm Mark's theory that this man had died and decomposed right on this very spot. The shaded, damp riverbank, inundated with new layers of silt each time the river flooded, was the perfect environ-ment for the creation of adipocere.

As soon as I knelt down beside the skull, however, I realized that my first impression had been wrong. This wasn't adipocere—it was lime.

That told me a whole different story. First of all, powdered lime doesn't appear naturally in the Kentucky woods. Somebody had to cart it all the way out here and sprinkle it over the dead man, to keep his body from smelling or to make it decompose more quickly. That didn't sound like a natural death to me.

Second, someone had had an awfully big stake in covering up this guy's death. By this point, I'd seen thousands of Kentucky homicide victims, and I could vouch for the fact that many people did very little to conceal their crimes. I'd seen a shocking number of girlfriends and family members who'd simply been killed and tossed into the woods. And since it's a felony to tamper with physical evidence, covering a body with lime added a second crime to the first one. Why had someone gone to so much trouble to hide this body?

Ironically, the lime intended to make the body disappear had actually helped preserve it. As soon as the river's moisture hit the lime's calcium carbonate, the powder had hardened, creating a crust that had encased our victim like a plaster-of-Paris shell. Only fragments of the lime remained. But when I lifted up the larger chunks of the hardened substance, I could see the reverse topography of a body, as if some perverse sculptor had used our victim's corpse to cast a mold.

When I called out that I had found lime, a shiver of anticipation ran through every cop at the scene as the implication of my words sank in. I knew we were all thinking the same thing: This was no accident. Thank heavens we had followed procedure and treated the area as a crime scene.

Now it was time to reach for the skull, and I was sorely tempted to simply snatch it from the soil and start checking for some sort of fatal injury. But I made myself go slowly. The detectives had pulled into a tight group above me on the riverbank, gazing down intently as I knelt over the half-buried skull, using a small soft-bristle paintbrush to brush away as much loose dirt and debris as I could. Then I followed the contours of the bone gently with my fingers, reaching as far into the soil as I dared, carefully lifting the skull from its resting place.

Breathless with anticipation, I turned the skull slowly in my hands. There was a neat round bullet hole directly behind the left ear, fractures radiating out from the hole like starbursts. Maybe tonight when I got home I'd feel some compassion for this man, shot in the head and left to rot in the dirt. Now all I felt was the thrill of the hunt.

Mark had come up behind me and was studying the skull over my shoulder. "Look," I said, tracing the bullet hole with my gloved finger.

"Here's an entrance gunshot wound. Now, do we have an exit wound, or have we gotten *really* lucky?" No exit wound might mean that the bullet itself was still inside the man's skull, an incredible piece of good fortune.

I turned the skull around slowly in my hand. Nope. No exit wound. The bullet that had killed this man might be lodged within these head bones, stuck inside the dirt and muck that over the years had taken the place of blood and brains.

Beside me, Mark was shaking his head, reluctant to give up his theory of a homeless man dead of natural causes. "Are you sure it's a bullet wound?" he asked stubbornly. "Maybe something here along the river bashed the skull after he died. Or maybe he just got drunk, fell down, and hit his head."

I heard a murmur of agreement from the officers higher up the bank. If this was a homicide, they'd have to find the killer. They needed to know what I thought and why I thought it. So, as I'd learned to do back in Tennessee, I started to think out loud, as much for my own benefit as for that of my colleagues.

"Okay," I began. "The first thing I do when I see a skull is to check for trauma. Hopefully, that tells me right off the bat whether we're looking at a homicide, suicide, or death from natural causes. If you're lucky enough to find a gunshot wound, that pretty much rules out natural causes. And depending on where the bullet hole is, you might be able to eliminate suicide or even accident."

I held up the skull a little higher, so everyone could see the hole. "Of course, you've got to be able to tell the difference between a gunshot wound and a hole that's been made in some other way. But see this beveling around the hole? To me, that spells 'bullet.' And look at these sharp fractures radiating out in all directions. You need speed and force to make fractures like that, so again, I'm thinking 'bullet.' "

"Okay, so it's not natural causes," Mark said reluctantly. "But what about suicide?"

"Or accidental death?" Daly chimed in. I could see him calculating all the different ways this investigation could go, wondering how much manpower he'd need, how much time.

"Check out the location of the wound," I suggested, pointing to the small, round hole about an inch behind where the victim's left ear used to be. "And look closely at the angle—the bullet was heading front and center. That's your classic execution-style gunshot wound. I'm not saying it couldn't have been an accident—but it's pretty unlikely. And no way was it suicide."

The men nodded and started to murmur among themselves. Violent crime was hardly a stranger to our fair Commonwealth. If we were going to discuss all the reasons a lone man might be found shot and buried in the woods, we'd be here until *next* Easter. So I left the police to their speculations and picked up my paintbrush again, using it to gently loosen some of the sandy soil from the skull's upper jaw and face area, holding the skull carefully over the small plastic box I'd brought for this purpose. As the grainy dirt fell into the box I thought about the intimate connection that had been created between this man's body and the sandy soil in which he'd been buried. His flesh had literally returned to dust—dust that I would later analyze back in my lab, hoping to find a bit of bone or bullet that might tell us who this man had been and who had killed him.

Once the skull's surface was relatively clean, I took a closer look at its grayish-brown contours. Years of work with Dr. Hughston and then in grad school had taught me to rely on my sense of touch, so I gently ran my fingers over the bones as if I were caressing the victim's face. I find this process totally mesmerizing, and I often catch myself slipping into a kind of trancelike state, in which I seem more open than usual to subtle impressions and unexpected insight.

To avoid becoming *too* absorbed, I make sure to keep up a running commentary, another thing I've learned the hard way. Once I had to examine a particularly large femur whose healed fracture up near the hip joint immediately caught my attention. As I wrapped my fingers gently around the bone and ran my hand up and down the shaft, the men around me all stopped what they were doing and gave me their full attention. I was oblivious of my audience until one of the detectives gently tapped me on the shoulder and asked in a stage whisper if I wanted to be alone. I laughed loudly with the others but I was mortified!

So now, I touched and talked at the same time, less concerned with whether the other investigators were listening than with identifying my own impressions. "Clearly, he was a man," I said, trying to keep my voice casual so I wouldn't sound *too* much like some fairground fortune-teller. "Big, robust face, very distinctive. Look at these heavy muscle markings—large facial features, for sure. He's got a big, prominent brow ridge, too. See this thick area of bone right above his eyes? When I first saw how big his skull was, I was pretty sure he was a male, but I know it now. Look at these big mastoid processes, the bones behind each ear. These were attached to the muscles that support and move the head; men usually have larger, stronger muscles than women."

I guess my audience was indeed listening, because a couple of them gave out a few good-natured cheers. I grinned at the interruption and went on to explain that since men's muscles are larger, all the places where their muscles are attached to bone tend to be larger, too. It's quite noticeable in the trunk, arms, and legs, but you can also see signs of maleness behind the ears and across the back of the skull.

As I reached the man's mid-face, my focus switched to our victim's racial heritage. His nose was long and narrow, with a fairly distinct sharp edge along the bottom, while the ridge of bone connecting the bottom of the nose to the upper teeth was almost vertical. At the top, both sides of the nose came together to form a narrow peak like a little tent, right between the skull's eye sockets. I could tell that this man's eyes had been set relatively close together, and that feature, plus his narrow nose, told me he'd probably had a significant amount of Caucasian ancestry. With the dirt and sand still stuck to the bone, it was difficult to form a specific opinion on his age, but judging by the overall maturity of his bones and teeth, he was clearly an adult.

When I took a closer look at our victim's teeth, I felt a surge of hope.

There was still a heavy veneer of dirt, but I could see that many teeth had been filled and covered with gold. Now we knew we were dealing with the homicide of an adult White male who could once afford the very best dental care available. After only two hours on the scene, this was progress.

Now, what about that bullet?

When you've got an entrance wound and no exit wound, the bullet is obviously going to lodge in the brain. In a fresh body, that's good news, because all you have to do is dissect it out either whole or in pieces if it's shattered inside the brain. As a body decomposes, however, the brain liquefies, and there's nothing to hold the bullet or its fragments in place. So it might easily slip out through one of the many large holes that once made room for the spinal cord, nerves, and arteries.

In this case, the cranial vault, or braincase, was packed full of silt. If we were lucky, this silt and sand had gradually filtered into the skull as the brain liquefied, trapping the bullet inside.

Mark had been watching closely as the other investigators gradually drifted back toward the perimeter of the crime scene, drinking their coffee and speculating further about who the dead guy might be. When I told him that we might still have the fatal bullet, his eyes lit up. "You know," he offered, "I've got an x-ray machine back at the office." Besides being the local coroner, Mark was a licensed chiropractor with an active practice in Fort Thomas. It could save us an awful lot of sifting and screening through the dirt.

"Sure," I agreed. "I'm done with the skull for now. Why don't you just pack it up and take it over to your office? We've got plenty to do till you get back."

Mark reached for the skull, but I couldn't help hesitating a bit before handing it over. I felt sure that he would indeed find the bullet, and to be honest, I was a little jealous. I couldn't decide whether to reassure myself that I might make an even bigger discovery than Mark, or to remind myself that after all, the end result was all that mattered. This question of who gets the credit had plagued me since my early days as a medical illustrator. I loved being part of a team, but I didn't like sitting anonymously on the bench. Well, I told myself, today I was not only part of the team, I was the star player, the captain, and the coach. The least I could do was let Mark score a point.

So, a little too much like a spoiled child giving up her favorite toy, I held out the skull, and eagerly Mark took it. Holding it upside-down in one hand, he climbed awkwardly back up the riverbank, where he meticulously wrapped the skull in a plastic bag. If the bullet was there, it wouldn't get far. And if it wasn't . . . I glanced at the choppy waters of the Ohio River and repressed a shudder. If the bullet that had killed this man had fallen out of his skull, we'd probably never see it again, though I was fully prepared to spend several hours sifting through the dirt to find it. "Leave those flags in place," I told my colleagues, pointing to the markers I'd put around the skull's original location. "And let's stay away from here for now." If we did have to dig for a bullet, I wanted to start with a relatively pristine section of soil.

Most of the man's bones had been partially freed from their clandestine grave by erosion, though they still lay half-buried under the sandy earth. Others perched precariously on chunks of sand that appeared ready to break off and slide into the river. I wondered how many days of floodwaters eating into the soil had finally freed these bones, and I marveled at the coincidence that had brought those two boys out here, after the bones had appeared but before they'd washed away for good.

Al interrupted my thoughts with a sharp tug on the safety rope. He had seen me maneuvering closer to the riverbank's crumbling brink, and he was taking no chances. I breathed a sigh of relief and waved up at him before kneeling once again beside the bones. I slowly repeated the careful, exacting procedure I had begun with the skull, gently brushing away loose dirt with a soft paintbrush, feeling for each bone's contours underground and then cautiously and patiently freeing it. Detective Lambers and I worked our way slowly but surely down to what should have been the victim's shoulders, brushing the silt and sand into plastic boxes, sealing the bones into labeled evidence bags, and passing our treasures up the riverbank, where other members of our team carefully catalogued each one.

There was a kind of hypnotic rhythm to our painstaking work, my hands moving on autopilot as my brain wandered off on its own. Something wasn't quite right about this case, but I couldn't figure out what it was. Then, as I gave a particularly vigorous tug to unloose the victim's shoulder blade, I realized what had been bothering me: the consistency of the dirt.

Any kid who's ever buried a toy or some secret treasure in the backyard knows that such objects are fairly easy to unearth a week or two later. After several months, though, the object gets packed in tighter. Something that's been buried for a year or more takes a fair amount of work to dislodge. Rain loosens the earth, and then gravity causes the loose particles to resettle themselves more tightly against the buried object. The object and the earth begin to bond, and with each passing year it becomes more difficult to separate the two, until the object seems almost to form part of the matrix within which it lies. At that point, you're not lifting out a discrete object—you're teasing out a piece of the whole.

That was the kind of work I'd been doing to free these bones, which told me that they'd been here far longer than the year or two I'd originally thought. I was starting to wonder exactly how long this man had been dead when I caught sight of something else I didn't expect—a bright metal object, lying just where the man's back hip pocket would have been.

I finished recovering the bone I'd been working on and turned my attention to the metal. With the same care I'd used for the bones, I managed to free the object, slowly but surely. Then I knelt there for a moment, staring at it in amazement. It was a thick, gold-colored money clip.

The heavy clip was layered with grime, but something about its weight and heft told me it had once been expensive. "Look at this," I said to Lambers, who shook his head.

"Not what you'd expect to find in some derelict's pocket, that's for sure."

I nodded. The man's gold fillings and expensive dental care had spoken of prosperity, but plenty of people fall on hard times. How likely was it, though, that a destitute man had a clip like this in his possession?

"Well, maybe he was a thief and had stolen it. But then, why didn't whoever killed him steal it from *him*?"

Lambers bagged and labeled the money clip, and passed it to the cop who stood above us. I heard the murmurs of surprise, the new rounds of speculation, follow the item up the bank. A moment later, we found a big pair of eyeglasses, scratched and worn, but still intact. And then a metal pen and pencil, heavy and corroded, like the money clip, still attached to the fabric that had once been this man's breast pocket. I couldn't tell through the dirt and grime, but it seemed to me that they, too, were gold-colored and part of a matching set, hinting, as the money clip did, at wealth.

As we worked our way down to the other hip and rear pocket area, we found a rusty lump of metal that had once been keys. Years of corrosion had fused them all together, and I couldn't wait to get them back to the lab and see what secrets they might hold. Then there was an old coin that I thought looked like a nickel, though it was so worn and dirty I couldn't be sure. Maybe it had a date on it, or some other clue that might point us toward this man's identity. A few minutes later, we found a second money clip, smaller and less elaborate than the first but with the same heavy, solid feel.

Throughout our excavation, I had also been freeing pieces of cloth from the silty earth, teasing them away from the ground as gently as I could. How long had it taken, I wondered, for the cloth to disintegrate into pieces? I was starting to get the distinct impression that these bones had lain here longer than any of us had suspected.

"Do you think that's a sheet?" Lambers asked, pointing at one swatch of fabric. While much of the cloth was the odd blue-green that Mark had first called workman's blue, this new piece of material seemed to have once been white.

I pulled the last corner of the cloth free and looked at its sagging folds. "Maybe a shirt?" I suggested. With the fabric all in pieces, it was hard to tell, but it seemed to me that this man had been dressed in a shirt—a fairly nice one, too, by the look of it—and some kind of business suit. Again, not what you'd expect from some homeless guy in the woods. I was becoming ever more intrigued by the emerging portrait of this man, his bones partially swathed in rotting cloth, his remains surrounded by his final earthly possessions like some Egyptian king laid out for burial. As we freed him and the objects around him from the fine-grained sandy soil, I felt that I was watching a long-forgotten photograph slowly come into focus, a moment frozen in time that was gradually making itself visible to my eyes.

I fingered a scrap of the dark-blue cloth, which seemed to be a well-worn synthetic. "Lucky he wasn't an all-natural guy," I murmured to Lambers. "Cotton or wool would be long gone by now."

"But what about the money clips?" Lambers asked. "And all the other stuff? Why didn't the killer take it? And Doc, how old is it?"

I shook my head. "Tomorrow," I said. I couldn't wait till we got this stuff back to the lab.

·   ·   ·

A few hours into the excavation, our safety-belt system was no longer working. As I continued to inch closer and closer to the crumbling edge of the riverbank, my legs were beginning to feel the strain of my constant balancing act, and I could only imagine how sore Al's arms were getting as he kept up his constant pull on my rope. The rest of our team was farther up the bank, but the photographer, videographer, and Lambers were right by my side as we migrated toward the dangerous drop-off.

The swollen Ohio had been rising steadily, its chilly waters now licking the edges of the bank about four feet below our ledge. With a certain amount of bravado, my three helpers had declined my offer of a safety rope. We had only one safety belt, and I was wearing it. My colleagues insisted that they were fine, but the safety officer called a halt. "Take a break, people!" he yelled down to us. "Help is on the way!"

I breathed a silent sigh of relief as I straightened my back and lay down my trowel. I could have used a break an hour ago, but surrounded by strong, fit cops, most of whom were decades younger than I was, I'd been reluctant to admit it. Sometimes I wonder just how long I can keep doing this type of strenuous fieldwork. I'm only in my midfifties, but I already use a walking stick, even while crossing level ground. One of the hazards of my profession is to make me all too uncomfortably conscious of how fragile my body is, holding me hostage to one torn ligament or pulled tendon, one bad twist of the knee or a sudden fall on the wrong part of my hip. Now I was extremely grateful for our half-hour enforced resting period before a local water rescue squad arrived at the scene: three men and a woman riding in a big flat-bottomed boat.

At first they simply stood by, ready to help if anyone should fall into the swift current, their boat bobbing in the choppy waters a few feet offshore. When they realized that the water was continuing to rise and the current was growing ever swifter, they jammed their bow right into the ledge, almost directly under my feet, their shoulders practically level with my hands. Suddenly, I had an idea.

"May I come on board?" I asked the rescue squad captain. He seemed a bit taken aback, but after a moment, he nodded yes. Still attached to my safety rope, I sat down in the dirt and slid down the exposed surface of the ledge until my feet were resting on the boat's bow. I carefully turned my head toward the ledge. Yes! I could excavate the rest of the site while standing in the boat. The site was just level with my chest, allowing me to hold my arms comfortably straight out in front of me.

With the help of one of the rescue squad, I unhooked my safety belt. "Heads up!" I called to the men on the shore, and tossed the belt up to Lambers, who put it on gratefully. We passed the next few hours in relative comfort, he wearing the belt, I standing in the boat.

Of course, there was one small problem: motion sickness. I probably could have handled the gentle rocking of the boat, but all day long huge barges kept making their majestic way up and down the Ohio, creating enormous wakes that rippled their way toward shore. Each time we collided with a wake, our boat would lurch, and I had to stop my work, standing stock-still, eyes squeezed shut, until the nausea passed. I must admit, it's the first time I ever got seasick while digging for a body.

·   ·   ·

Mark still hadn't gotten back from his office, and I was starting to get worried about losing the bullet, especially now that bits of soil had started to crumble away from the bank, so my gallant rescue crew improvised a solution. Two men held a wooden backboard up against the bank, allowing me to examine the loose fragments of earth before they fell into the river and were gone forever. I didn't mind the dirt, but I was taking no chances on losing our bullet.

My patience was starting to wear thin, though. "Where is Dr. Schweitzer?" I asked at about two in the afternoon, and as if on cue Mark came running over the hill waving a large brown envelope.

"I've got the x-rays!" he called down to us. "I can see the bullet in his skull!" This was certainly a welcome bit of news, though I had to laugh at how my earlier envy had melted into relief. It was good to know that when push came to shove, I really was more interested in getting the results than in taking the credit.

When Mark made his careful way down to the ledge, I pointed to the large tree root I had just unearthed. "Look, Mark. This actually grew right into his pants. It got inside his pants leg through a small hole near the hip, then grew parallel to his thigh bone for years."

Mark looked more closely at the root, which was several inches in diameter. "How long do you think he's been there?" he asked in an awed whisper.

I shook my head. The bones felt old to me, and the associated evidence—the cloth and objects unearthed along with the bones—had clearly been in the ground for quite a while. In my own mind, I was saying, Ten years? Twenty? But until I could get everything to the lab, I was taking no chances on committing to the wrong answer, even to myself. This case had already thrown us more than its share of curve-balls, and I wanted to keep an open mind.

·   ·   ·

Lambers and I had agreed that he'd maintain the evidence overnight, bringing it to my lab first thing the next morning. Like a nervous host-ess, I scurried around the lab, hurrying to clear away the skeletal remains and paperwork from the case I'd been working on the week before. I'd just doused the counters with disinfectant and loaded my favorite Patsy Cline CD into the stereo when Lambers arrived, look-ing very much like an overburdened shopper as he clutched several big brown bags tightly to his chest, the inventory list tucked under his chin.

"Come on, Doc," he said without moving his jaw, as I rushed to take his burdens from him. "Where should we get started?"

I smiled at his enthusiasm and couldn't help thinking that he, at least, seemed no worse for wear after yesterday's efforts. I wasn't about to tell him that I was stiff and sore.

"Let's start with the skull," I suggested. "I can't wait to get my hands on that bullet." Lambers watched in fascination as I soaked the skull in a basin of water, rinsing all the dirt away. Then I set up a fine wire-mesh screen, poured the dirty water through it, and breathed a sigh of triumph. There lay the bullet, intact upon the screen.

I took a picture of the bullet and packed it carefully into a small envelope labeled with the case number, the date, and my initials. Later I'd take it downstairs to the ballistic experts in the state police lab.

Lambers and I looked at the rest of the evidence bags, feeling like two kids on Christmas morning. So much intriguing evidence—where would we begin?

"There's no real way to decide," I said finally. "Let's just pick what interests us most and start there."

Lambers nodded and said exactly what I was thinking: "The money clip."

As I went through the shopping bags, Lambers prepared to resume his job from the day before, taking notes on everything I said and did. With mounting excitement, I pulled out the two plastic evidence bags that held the money clips. Even through the sand and ground-in dirt, I could see that the larger one was engraved with an intricate cross-hatch pattern and the initials HS—or was it SH? Frustratingly, both ways looked correct. The other one was engraved also, but with simple straight lines. Both bore marks indicating they were made of 14-karat gold.

Lambers was quick to conclude that this probably wasn't a robbery. "These were in his pockets, Doc. It's hard to believe that someone would take a wad of bills out of solid-gold money clips and then put the clips back into the guy's pocket."

I had to agree. "And you can't quite see some derelict just picking them up while scrounging around, can you? You'd need a wad of bills to buy each one."

I took the clips over to my sink and gently rinsed them in clear, warm water, removing the last traces of sand with a soft toothbrush. After I laid them on a clean blue towel to dry, Lambers and I each took several photographs with both conventional and digital cameras. In this case, Lambers and I would rely on conventional photographs as evidence, but I e-mailed the electronic pictures to Detective Daly in Fort Thomas, where they appeared on the evening news that very night.

Next, I looked at the eyeglasses, their cloudy lenses surrounded with thick black plastic frames. "Not too stylish, are they?" I asked Lambers, who was busy noting the time I had opened the bag.

"No, but they sure are big." Indeed they were: From side to side, the earpieces measured almost eight inches.

"Well, his bones are big," I answered. "And with these glasses, it looks like a lot of flesh must have covered his bones, but we'll know more once we get to his clothes. That's going to be a monumental task, so let's say we do a few more easy ones first." Lambers nodded as he handed me the bag labeled SOCKS.

The socks were made of a thin synthetic fiber and were almost twenty inches long, another indication that our victim had been large. At the top of each cuff, I found a clump of rusty metal imbedded in the fabric. When I scraped off the corrosion with a small knife, I saw that these were garter snaps. This man had been wearing knee socks, held up by garters—an unusual style, to say the least.

Lambers handed me the bag labeled GLOVES. They were big, too, but I could see that they'd been hand-stitched from smooth leather. The same was true of his belt.

Now I couldn't wait to get a good look at his clothes. Although Mark had originally described the cloth as workman's blue, it was actually closer to a dark blue-green. As I carefully pulled the fragile fabric from the evidence bag, I brushed off the loose dirt, flattened the fabric with my hands, and laid it out on the gurney. Soon I could see that each piece was an individual panel of the same garment. The threads that once held these garments together had disintegrated, perhaps because, until the last few decades, most thread was made of cotton, a natural fiber that decomposes rapidly. The cloth itself was in remarkably good shape. It looked and felt like polyester, a petroleum-based product that theoretically can last forever.

After an hour's careful unfolding and matching, I managed to reassemble a pair of trousers, a suit jacket, and a long-sleeved shirt. As I looked at his clothes, I began to imagine the man who had worn them had been a large, heavyset man. Fat? Or perhaps he'd just been big-boned and well-muscled. So far, all we knew was that he'd worn big clothes. A simple measuring tape told us that his jacket measured 58 inches around the chest, while it had taken a 48-inch waistband to circle his waist. His arms and his legs were long, and his neck was big too, almost 18 inches in circumference.

Although the threads connecting these panels were gone, I could still see the seams and darts, and it appeared as if the suit had been hand-tailored to a custom fit. Evidently, he'd been stylishly dressed, but for what era? After we'd finished recovering all these things yesterday, I would have guessed that they'd lain in their secret grave for at least ten years. But I associated this type of tailored polyester suit with the mid-1960s. (Lambers, of course, had never seen one at all!)

"This guy dresses like a Cold-War Russian," I found myself saying, and then asked myself what had brought that image to mind. Something in the cut of his suit recalled for me TV footage of foreign dignitaries meeting with President John F. Kennedy, something old-fashioned and European. . . .

I pulled out a pencil and a couple of sheets of paper and tapped into my rusty medical-illustration skills. As Lambers called out the measurements of each garment, I sketched out labeled diagrams of the suit jacket, the trousers, and the shirt, complete with notes about the placement and size of buttons, pockets, pleats, even the epaulets on the shoulders of the shirt, and not forgetting the type and manufacturer of the zipper. As Lambers watched in fascination, I went online to search vintage clothing sites.

I showed him a few images. "What do you think?" I asked him. "1960s? 1970s? We're getting back there, anyway."

Lambers shook his head. "If he was killed way back then, we'll never find out who did it."

I sighed. "Right now I'm more concerned with figuring out who he was."

"That won't be easy either."

He was right, of course. It was hard enough identifying a pile of bones that had lain in the woods for a year or more. If this man had been there for two or three decades . . .

"Anyway, the clothes give us somewhere to start," I said. I shot off a few e-mails to the names I'd seen on the vintage clothing sites we'd just browsed. An expert opinion might at least pinpoint the year these clothes had been in fashion. That wouldn't be definitive—the victim might have stolen the clothes, or borrowed them, or bought them from a thrift shop. He might even be the kind of guy who wore the same suit for decades. But, as I'd told Lambers, it was a place to start.

We moved on to the gold pen and pencil set. When I gently scraped away the dirt from the pen's clip, I began to make out a faint logo: C-R-O-S-S.

"It's a Cross pen," I said to Lambers. I could tell by his blank look that the name meant nothing. "Cross," I repeated. "It's a kind of upscale brand. For people who care about that kind of thing, it's maybe the Rolls-Royce of pens. Each one of them is individually made, and all by hand. A friend of mine wanted to get one for her nephew's graduation, and she only spent about a hundred dollars, but she told me that some models cost more than five hundred."

Lambers's eyes widened. "For a *pen?*"

I pointed to the next evidence bag. "And a pencil. Solid gold, matching set . . ." I made a mental note to contact the Cross company. Maybe they could tell me when this particular style had been on the market.

I was eager to get on to the keys and the coin, but it would take hours to clean off the corrosion that had been building up over the years, and I was even more eager to look at the bones. By now, my examining room was crammed full of gurneys stacked with evidence, notepaper, and cameras, so I set to clearing some space while Lambers finished with his notes and pictures. Once again my hands went on autopilot while my mind roamed free. I could almost see our victim now: a wealthy man, well dressed in a business suit, leather gloves, and knee socks with garters. He had a faintly European air, and he carried himself like a man who was used to the best: a monogrammed money clip, a gold Cross pen and pencil set. For some reason, he'd gone or been taken down to an isolated spot on the banks of the Ohio. And there was something else: Someone had held a gun to his skull and pulled the trigger.

By now I'd moved all the other evidence onto the counters lining the periphery of the lab, and I was ready to start with the bones. As I took each one out of its evidence bag, I laid it out on the gurney, so that a disarticulated skeleton gradually emerged. I finally added the skull and mandible. Our guy's face and jaws were still covered in debris from the grave, but I knew from yesterday's quick field exam that he'd had several gold crowns and fillings in his mouth. The x-rays that Mark had taken yesterday had revealed more fillings, bright white spots on the film that were the same density as the bullet.

Now, as I carefully brushed away the sand, mud, and traces of lime, I was treated to another welcome surprise. These teeth had not only been crowned and filled with gold, they'd been extremely clean and well cared for, with no evidence of active decay at the time of death.

"This was no derelict," I told Lambers. "He had money right up until he died." So far, we might have been dealing with someone who'd once been wealthy but who had gone on to face hard times. I'd seen many such cases before: a man who becomes destitute after years of comfortable living; the daughter of wealthy parents who pay for her expensive composite fillings only while she lives at home. You see signs of expensive dental care, yes, but you can also read the hard times that came later: the cavities, the buildup of tartar and calculus, the gum disease. You might even notice a missing tooth or two.

Not with this guy. Although decades of chewing had ground down the surfaces of his teeth a little, he had maintained a nice smile until the day he died—a nice, expensive smile.

I looked more closely at the man's skull, trying to imagine his face. His head was large and well rounded, with a square jaw that fit well into the temporomandibular joint, the place where the mandible attaches to the skull. That joint showed no signs of arthritis, so he'd had no trouble chewing with those well-kept teeth. The bridge of his nose was formed by exceptionally large, prominent nasal bones. I pictured a big protruding nose, and then a huge forehead, the flesh jutting out to cover the heavy brow ridge. He'd have had a rugged, masculine face, with well-proportioned features and a sparkling smile. Judging by the clothes he'd worn, he'd had a significant amount of flesh covering these big bones. I noticed the well-defined muscle insertions, which usually indicate big, strong muscles. He was probably a hefty guy, but not fat. More meaty, like a wrestler. Or maybe a football player?

Lambers was getting restless. After all, we already knew that this man was a large White male. What else could the bones tell us? I decided to go back to my thinking-out-loud method, so Lambers could share in my search.

"So far, I haven't seen any old fractures, but the ends of the long bones and the lower spine had started to show some wear. Those teeth of his had worn down a little too, so I think we could bump his age up into the forty-to-fifty-five range." I wanted to narrow that down, but it'd have to do for the moment. "Now, let's see how tall this guy was." I opened a cabinet and pulled out a giant set of sliding calipers.

In spite of himself, Lambers was intrigued. "What are you going to do, Doc? Connect all these bones and measure from top to bottom?"

"Luckily, I don't have to. I'm just going to measure his thigh bone and then ask the computer here to figure out the rest." Anthropologists before my time made great progress in estimating stature by using mathematical formulas and statistical analyses. These formulas have recently been computerized and bolstered by data from modern forensic cases, so now all I had to do was type in the femur measurement. A computer program called FORDISC 2.0 would do the rest.

I laid the man's femur flat on the counter, placing one straight flat needle of the caliper against the bottom side of the knee and the other against the rounded ball at the top. Most anthropologists use an osteometric board to take these measurements; it resembles a fish-measuring board, or one of those devices that measures your foot at the shoe store, but I find that a caliper is just as accurate and much more efficient, especially when the bones in question are still covered with flesh. The osteometric board only works on free-standing bones, but I can insert the needles of my calipers into the joints and ends of bones that are still attached to a body.

This femur was 536 millimeters long. When FORDISC 2.0 learned that these measurements had belonged to a White male, it obligingly reported a height of 6 feet, 4 inches, give or take a few inches.

"He was huge," remarked Lambers, who looked about 5'10" at most.

"I'm 5'8"." I nodded in agreement at him before looking at my sketch of the suit. "Yeah, he was pretty bulky. But given how tall he was, I don't think he was roly-poly fat, just big all over. I'd say he weighed close to 250 pounds. So when we start going through missing persons files, we can knock out the short, skinny guys immediately."

Identifying this man was everybody's top priority at the moment. News of our discovery had hit the airwaves all over northern Kentucky and southern Ohio, and my voice mail was already clogged with messages from reporters. Luckily, departmental protocol wouldn't let me talk to the press this early in the process; I could only discuss this case with the coroner and the detective in charge. So I called Mark and Detective Daly and told them what we'd learned. We all knew it was crucial to capitalize on this narrow window of opportunity while the press and the public were still interested.

Mark and Daly listened eagerly as I ran down our discoveries. Then Daly asked the one question I couldn't answer: "How long do you think he's been dead?"

As I'd done yesterday, I shook my head. "It's been a while, I'll say that much. Twenty years? Twenty-five? Let's keep it vague for now. Maybe tomorrow I'll find out more."

•　　　•　　　•

The next morning there was an e-mail message waiting for me from Daphne Harris, proprietor of the Red Rose Vintage Clothing Company in Indianapolis. To my amazement, she had answered me right away, estimating that the suit I'd sketched had been made sometime between 1955 and 1963. I immediately sent her pictures of the eyeglasses and the monogrammed money clip, and her answers were similar: 1955 to 1965 for the glasses, and the 1940s or 1950s for the clip.

Well, that at least gave us a back date. But maybe this guy was just old-fashioned. Or maybe he was wearing someone else's stuff, though I couldn't think of a reason why he'd do that. I was longing for a more precise date of death, but I knew we'd been incredibly lucky to get as much as we had. If all we'd had was the bones, we'd have been stuck.

By this time, local and state police agencies had already searched their missing persons files, and they had no records matching my description. That wasn't surprising for a case that was at least two decades old. It was even less surprising for this particular corner of Kentucky, which had been a lawless center of illegal gambling and prostitution from the 1930s through the 1960s. The Cleveland Syndicate, a Mafia-related crime ring heavily into gambling, had moved in right after the end of World War II and had remained in control until the 1960s, when U.S. Attorney General Robert Kennedy and his colleagues began lengthy investigations into the problem and backed political reformers in the whole region, including Campbell County.

When I took another look at the dates and thought about the organized crime connection, a wild thought came to mind. Was it possible that this rich man, executed decades ago and encased in lime, was actually Jimmy Hoffa? After all, the money clip read either HS or SH, what if the H stood for Hoffa? I knew it was a wild hunch, but my fingers trembled as I called my colleagues at the FBI.

They soon put an end to that theory. Hoffa's missing person's report, they told me, identified him as 5'5" and 180 pounds. He was clearly way too short and thin to be our guy.

Meanwhile, I was reaching out to experts across the country. I sent the pen and pencil to the A. T. Cross Company in Lincoln, Rhode Island, hoping they could tell me when the items were manufactured. I sent the coin—it *was* a nickel—to the U.S. Mint, hoping that they could tell me whether the little date on the bottom really was 1964. (The coin was so corroded, I couldn't be sure.) The eyeglasses went to a local optical company to see if they could find any clues hidden in the frame style or the prescription. I took the skull to Dr. Mark Bernstein, our consultant in forensic odontology. And I sent the clothes and the money clips to the Fort Thomas Police Department for safe-keeping.

One week after our trip to the river, all that remained in my lab were the bones and the keys. I'd gotten all I could from the bones. It was time to look at the keys.

•   •   •

The keys were a solid mass, fused together by years of corrosion. At first I thought I could simply pry them apart, and I did manage to break away two of the outer keys. The third time was definitely not the charm, however: The key split right down the middle. I'd have to find a better approach.

I laid out a piece of white butcher paper on my lab counter, then pulled out some petri dishes and a jar of naval jelly. Naval jelly is an acid that was originally used to remove rust and corrosion from metal objects such as ships, hence its name. I thought that at the very least I could use it to separate the keys. What I really hoped for was to read a manufacturer's name and city, but first things first.

I soaked the keys in the naval jelly for about an hour, then rinsed them in clear water to remove the acid. I was walking a fine line: I wanted the acid to eat away the corrosion while leaving intact any writing or logos on the keys. By alternately soaking and rinsing over a period of about two days, I was able to separate the rest of the keys without breaking any more of them.

The individual keys were still corroded, however, and no writing was visible to the naked eye. Full of optimism, I examined each one through my dissecting microscope. Yes, indeed I could just barely make out a cluster of tiny letters, stamped around the edge of two of the keys.

The letters were scarcely legible, but I thought that making them more three-dimensional might make them easier to read. So I turned off the room lights and worked under the single light of a freestanding halogen lamp, which had been positioned to hit each key at an angle. When I looked at a key under a large wall-mounted magnifying glass, I could see the contours of each letter on it a little more clearly. And when I delicately scraped each key's stamped surface with the blade of a scalpel, I managed to remove the decades-long corrosion a fraction of a millimeter at a time. Finally, I could read the secrets of the keys.

What I found sent me hurrying to the phone. After several long-distance calls, I dialed one final number.

Detective Daly picked up the phone. "I hope you're sitting down," I told him. "Because you're not going to believe this. Our John Doe is from Connecticut."

I could feel his surprise even over the phone. "What makes you say that, Doc?" he said finally.

"The keys were made by Connecticut locksmiths. One is imprinted with the words DEPIERNE, NORWALK, CONN. and one reads KARPELOW SAFE AND LOCK. I can even read a partial address on that one." I couldn't read it all, but I had managed to make out a few key letters and numbers: _82 ELM STREET, _____PORT, CT. When I called the U.S. Post Office, they told me that those two-letter state designations were implemented in 1963. So the Karpelow key might have been made any time after 1963, and the DePierne key was imprinted no later than 1963, maybe earlier.

Daly's reaction was all I could have hoped for. "Doc, this is *huge*," he said hoarsely. "Let me make some calls, and I'll get back with you as soon as I know something."

Early the next morning, he called back. "Okay, we've narrowed down the time just a bit more. Seems DePierne went out of business about twenty-five years ago, and Karpelow moved from that Elm Street address back in the 1970s."

From that point on, the investigation took on a life of its own as the answers to the previous week's questions started pouring in. The Cross company told me that the particular model of pen and pencil I'd sent them had been made only between 1965 and 1970. The nickel did indeed bear the date of 1964. The eyeglasses had most likely been made during that same era in either Japan or Germany, which might help to explain my European imagery. And although he described the dental work much more clinically in his report, Dr. Bernstein told me that in his opinion, the teeth in our guy's mouth looked like expensive Park Avenue dentistry at its finest.

Then, on May 25, Daly called me at home a little after dinner. As soon as I heard his voice I knew he had exciting news, otherwise he'd have waited till the next day. "Do you feel lucky?" he asked me. He started to chuckle, then laughed out loud. "I had a reporter, Mike Mayko, run a piece about our John Doe in the *Connecticut Post,* and I just now spoke with him. He has a tip for us that came in through their crime stoppers hotline."

A wealthy businessman had apparently disappeared from Weston, Connecticut, on March 25, 1966, right after he'd made an appearance before a New York City grand jury. This man had been one of three people accused of conspiring to evade $7 million in taxes owed on foreign stock trades. He'd reportedly left his home around 4:00 p.m. in a 1965 green Corvette Stingray and boarded an American Airlines flight from Kennedy Airport to Cincinnati under the assumed name of Mr. Henry. Then he simply vanished.

"Now here's the best part," Daly told me. "The man's name is Henry Scharf."

"Oh, my God. The initials on the money clip. So they *were* H.S. That's got to be him. Was he as big as I estimated?"

"You were right on target about everything. Mayko told me the guy was really tall and built like a pro football player. Obviously, he had money. He was 46 when he disappeared. And remember those German eyeglass frames? This guy traveled regularly to France and Germany."

Now it was my turn to be stunned.

"So," Daly went on, "I've got a Connecticut detective working on the next step. The tipster who saw the article in the paper, though, said contacting the family might not be too easy. He knows them, and they were so devastated by the incident that they may not want to have anything to do with the police."

"But that was almost thirty years ago," I said without thinking. "They have to be ready to talk about it now." I couldn't stand the idea of being so close and then losing all hope of identification, especially for such a sad reason: decades of unhealed bitterness.

"First things first," Daly told me. "Let me talk to them."

As it turned out, the Scharf family was reluctant to talk to the police, but they were willing to talk to me. Perhaps a scientist or a doctor seemed less threatening to them than someone in law enforcement. When I spoke with Henry's son-in-law, who was acting as the spokesman for his wife and mother-in-law, I could tell that the wounds were still fresh, a quarter-century later, but the family was being as cooperative as they could be.

Then we ran into a different kind of problem. Because of the time lag, nothing was falling into place. Mrs. Scharf didn't recognize the money clips. Henry's dentist had died years ago, and his inactive records had been destroyed. (I couldn't help feeling pleased to learn that he actually *was* from Park Avenue!) Henry had had fingerprints on file with the FBI, but the skin was long gone from our victim's phalanges. Although Henry had been in the U.S. Army, his medical and dental records had been destroyed when a fire had ripped through the military archives in St. Louis.

Undaunted, I asked the family for a photograph, and they sent one that showed a robust, smiling Henry standing on a boat, holding up a large fish. To my artist's and anthropologist's eyes, it looked like a match to John Doe's skull. Now I was personally convinced that we had found the remains of Henry Scharf. But I still had to prove it.

Then I got what I thought was another break. With the help of the U.S. Department of Veterans Affairs, I discovered that Henry had filed a claim for benefits, which had left a dental chart on file with the department. With help from the FBI, I got a copy of this chart and set about comparing it to the teeth in the victim's skull.

They didn't match.

No. It wasn't possible. I *knew* the chart had to be wrong. But how could I explain the discrepancy? The chart indicated that Henry was missing a molar. That same molar was present in the skull I held in my hand.

I decided that the dentist had simply made a mistake, and with more bravado than brains, I ignored the dental chart. "Let's do a DNA comparison," I told Mark and Detective Daly. "At this point, we've got to know."

I guess Mark and Daly were as eager as I was to know the truth, because they eventually agreed. But a DNA analysis wouldn't be easy. DNA analysis is based upon the premise that every cell of our bodies contains a genetic code, identical throughout our bodies and highly similar to the codes found among our close relatives. In theory, then, any cell from any body can be used to do a comparative DNA analysis.

When living people or fresh bodies are involved, this process is relatively easy. You use the DNA found in a cell's nucleus, but nucleic DNA is quite fragile and cannot withstand the ravages of time. So when long-dead bodies are involved, another part of the cell must be invaded to extract the more durable mitochrondrial DNA, a tedious and expensive process.

Extraction is only half the problem. Mitochondrial DNA is only inherited from the mother. So it must be compared to the blood of a relative within the maternal lineage.

Then we got our final and most important break. We found out that Henry Scharf's sister was still alive.

· · ·

"Mrs. Greenberg?"

After delicate negotiations with members of Henry's extended family, I had been granted permission to speak with Henry's sister, Minna Greenberg (not her real name). Henry's niece had told her mother that Henry's body had been found, and Mrs. Greenberg knew I'd had something to do with that. But this eighty-year-old woman knew very little else, only that her beloved brother had mysteriously disappeared well over a quarter of a century ago, leaving his family bereft.

It wasn't the first tragedy Minna had suffered. In 1939, she and her brother had fled Austria in the wake of the Nazi invasion. As Jews, they were eager to leave, though they'd had to leave behind a large number of loved ones. Although Minna had eventually lost everyone except her beloved brother, she had never given up hope until now.

"So, you're the one who found my dear Henry." Her voice was quavering but surprisingly strong, her Austrian accent still evident.

"I was one of the people who helped find him, yes." I'd never had a conversation like this before. Usually it's the police and the coroners who talk to the survivors. "At least, I think we've found him. That's why we need your help." I told her what we knew and what we didn't know.

"And what do you need from me?"

I explained about the DNA test, my voice hesitant as I stumbled over the words. In her place, I'd want to know for sure, even thirty-four years later. But perhaps she preferred not to know. Or maybe she'd spun out some fantasy of Henry living happily, safely, somewhere else, unable, for some inexplicable reason, to tell his family where he was. Maybe she didn't want closure. Maybe, having lost so many others, she preferred to keep this door open.

After I finished talking, there was a long pause. I searched wildly for something else to say, something that might convince her or maybe just something that would bring her comfort. But before I could say anything, Minna spoke.

"All right," she said simply. "You can have some of my blood. How do we proceed?"

The final arrangements were made with the help of the FBI. A sample of Minna's blood was taken in Florida and flown to LabCorp in North Carolina, where the mitochondrial DNA was compared to a sample from a bone of our victim.

It was a match.

.   .   .

The rest of the puzzle remains maddeningly incomplete. Why had
Henry flown to Cincinnati? What was his connection (if any) to the
Cleveland Syndicate? Why had he been killed? When I think back on
the case of Henry Scharf, I sometimes see it as my greatest triumph.
Identifying a victim who's been dead and hidden for over thirty years
is an extremely rare achievement. Yet if it's a triumph, it's an extremely
frustrating one, my happy memories of discovering the bullet and reading the keys intermixed with the heart-wrenching thought of that final
phone call. I would have liked to have given Minna Greenberg the satisfaction of telling her who had killed her brother and why. But maybe,
after everything else she'd been through, just knowing that he hadn't
willingly deserted her was enough.

6

Finding Names for the Dead

Bereavement in their death to feel
Whom we have never seen—
A vital kinmanship import
Our souls and theirs between.

— EMILY DICKINSON

O KAY, GUYS, I MADE IT. We're going to start digging now." I
was trying to sound positive, but my voice rang hollow, even
to me.

"Don't get too comfortable down there, Doc. We still have to haul
you out."

I looked at the dirt walls surrounding me and shook my head. I was
standing literally at the bottom of a grave, on a gray, freezing, late-
winter day. Comfort was not an option.

I don't participate in all that many exhumations, but even if I had, this one would have been special. We were trying to recover the buried bones of the "Tent Girl," a mysterious young woman whose remains had been found some thirty years ago.

I'd first learned of Tent Girl only a few days after I'd taken the job as state forensic anthropologist. Scott County Coroner Marvin Yokum had come to me with Tent Girl's picture, explaining that this was a case that had gone unsolved for decades.

It all started on the morning of May 17, 1968, when an unemployed well-driller living in Monterey, Kentucky, was out looking for old glass telephone insulators, which he used to sell for extra money. That morning, as he searched through the underbrush around Eagle Creek, he stumbled over an old green tarpaulin tied with a small thin cord. Inside the tarp were the badly decomposed remains of a naked young woman with a piece of white fabric wrapped around her head.

Marvin took charge. His autopsy report eventually described the woman as sixteen to nineteen years old, 5'1" tall, weighing 110–115 pounds, with short, reddish-brown hair. A pathologist brought in from nearby Hamilton County, Ohio, told Marvin that the young woman had probably been wrapped up in the canvas, bound, and left to die, slowly, of suffocation.

The investigation had gone on for months, and Marvin had even called in the FBI. The Bureau had managed to determine that the white cloth was probably a diaper, but found very little else that could be used to identify her. When the local newspaper ran a story on the victim, they called her Tent Girl, because of the canvas tarp. The paper had asked Covington police officer Harold Musser for sketches based on the autopsy photos, and something about the wistful young woman with her waifishly short hair caught the public's imagination. When Tent Girl was finally laid to rest in the Georgetown Cemetery—only a few miles from where I now live—the marker on her grave read simply "#90"—the number of her anonymous plot.

Three years later, two men who owned a local monument company built her a special headstone—red, to match her hair—with a version of the sketch etched into the granite. The Tent Girl became a local legend, drawing visitors from all over Kentucky and Ohio, especially young women, who seemed to feel a special kinship with her.

Marvin felt something for her, too, and when I took the job in Kentucky he thought he saw a fresh chance of solving a case that had bothered him for years. He brought me the autopsy photos and Musser's sketches, and asked if I could maybe do a better sketch. However, to my artist's and anthropologist's eye, the sketch artist had done an excellent job. He'd been true to all the scientific detail available in the photo—and, somehow, he'd made the young woman's face come alive.

"I honestly don't think I could improve on these," I told Marvin. "The problem isn't with the sketches. The problem is that the right person hasn't seen them yet."

Marvin was reluctant to accept this, but I'd seen it already in my short career and I'd have cause to see it again throughout the years. Facial reconstructions are basically a shot in the dark. If you're lucky enough to get the right person to see them, they work. If you're not, they don't. The quality of the facial reconstruction is important, sure, but that alone won't bring you success. Luck has a lot more to do with it.

And, indeed, it was luck that had brought me here today. Some thirty years after Tent Girl had been laid to rest, I was standing in her grave—because someone finally thought he knew who she was.

"Do you have enough room over there, Doc?" My grave-digging companion, a local deputy, was standing right beside me, trying not to step on any of the bones. We'd excavated the grave with a backhoe, but the young woman had been buried without a coffin, so as soon as we caught sight of the first bone, I'd climbed down into the hole. Now I was on my knees with a hand trowel, recovering those few bones that hadn't long ago crumbled into earth. Later that week, we would try to match their mitochondrial DNA with the blood of someone who thought that Tent Girl might be her long-lost sister.

The deputy was standing ready with a shovel, prepared to toss out the dirt that I dug up. "Seems to me like you've got all the hard work," I told him, scraping a little more soil away from the half-buried fibula. "This looks like the easy part to me."

He shook his head. "I'm just as happy not to have to dig up a dead woman's bones," he said. "I'll leave that little job to you."

.   .   .

The story of how Tent Girl's identity had finally been discovered was one that would make even the most arrogant investigator bow her head and give thanks for the dedicated efforts of interested civilians. Some twenty years after that well-driller had found the body, he'd moved to Livingston, Tennessee, where his daughter, Lori, started dating a seventeen-year-old boy named Todd Matthews. Todd hadn't even been born when Lori's father found the Tent Girl, but something about the anonymous young woman caught his imagination. Todd went on to marry Lori and his interest in Tent Girl increased, almost to the point of obsession. Eventually, he made it his life's work to discover Tent Girl's identity.

Todd's all-consuming interest in the case began to threaten his marriage and drastically cut into the time he spent with his own young son. When he realized that the Internet could significantly expand his ability to search for clues, he started spending hour after hour at his computer. Late one night in January 1998, after his wife and child had gone to bed, Todd clicked on to a missing persons website—and struck pay dirt. There was a description of a young woman who had gone missing from Lexington, Kentucky. Somehow, intuitively, Todd knew that this was the woman he sought.

The description had been posted by Rosemary Westbrook, a forty-year-old woman then living in Arkansas. Rosemary's father and brother had been killed by floods in Illinois two weeks before she was born, and her mother's hands were full caring for the other six children. Baby Rosemary was sent to live with relatives who made sure she kept in close touch with her mother, brothers, and sisters.

When she was ten, Rosemary learned that her older sister Barbara Ann Hackmann Taylor, then twenty-four, had mysteriously disappeared. As an adult, Rosemary decided that she wanted to find her missing sister. The previous August, she had posted a description of Barbara—the very posting Todd Matthews found that January night:

Name: Barbara Ann (Hackmann) Taylor
Relationship: Sister
Date of Birth: 9-12-1943
Female

Remarks: My sister Barbara has been missing from our family since the latter part of the year 1967. She has brown hair, brown eyes, around 5 feet, 2 inches tall, last seen in the Lexington, Kentucky, area. If you have any information on my sister, please contact me at the address posted.

When Todd called Rosemary and gave her the details about the Tent Girl, she, too, became convinced that this was her missing sister, known to family and friends as Bobbie. Apparently Bobbie had married a man named George Earl Taylor, with whom she'd traveled the carnival circuit in the mid-1960s. When Bobbie disappeared, George took their baby son and daughter to live with his parents, telling them that Bobbie had run off with a trucker. The son had died as a young adult, but the surviving daughter was still haunted by the knowledge that her mother had never come back to get her, had never sent so much as a postcard to say she remembered her child.

Bobbie had also helped raise George's daughter from a previous marriage. That daughter later told Rosemary that she'd last seen Bobbie in Lexington, Kentucky—a detail that made Todd more certain than ever that Tent Girl was Barbara Ann Hackmann Taylor. He contacted Marvin Yokum, who after all these years was still Scott County coroner.

Once again, Marvin and I met in my office, along with Scott County Detective John Ferris. This time, besides Tent Girl's autopsy photos, Marvin was able to show me photos of Barbara Ann.

In the first one, she looked somber, her mouth closed, her eyes serious as she stared into the camera. I looked slowly back and forth between that forty-year-old photograph and the old sketch of Tent Girl. Yes, I thought. Everything looked right—the proportions of the features, the shape of the face. This could be a match.

"Do you have any other pictures?" I asked.

Marvin slid another photograph across my desk, a three-quarter view in which Bobbie's mouth was open just a little, exposing a couple of teeth. I looked closely at the autopsy photo that had been taken of the decomposed head and face and noticed several similarities. I couldn't see enough teeth in Bobbie's picture to be absolutely certain, but maybe—just maybe—it was a match.

"It's not enough for a positive ID, though," I added quickly, and saw Marvin's look of disappointment. "First of all, the photograph's too fuzzy. And secondly, the teeth just aren't that unusual. I mean, if you get a real clear picture with someone's mouth open real wide, and maybe the person has a gold front tooth with a heart carved in it, or if a tooth is totally rotated and then the one next to that is missing—then, yes, a forensic odontologist can make a positive ID from that." I gestured toward the snapshot lying on my desk, one of those Kodak specials from forty years ago, with the white border and the little date stamped on it. "This is so close, though, I think we can justify looking at DNA."

Marvin nodded. "All right then," he said finally. "I think we've got to dig up her grave."

Detective Ferris and I agreed that an exhumation and DNA comparison were warranted. We, too, were eager to solve the mystery of the Tent Girl, who had become such a big part of local legend. But it was still the middle of winter, and the ground was frozen solid. Although the coroner soon got the exhumation order from the state officials, it would be weeks before the weather cleared enough for us to use it.

Then, one day, I heard on the radio that the temperature was supposed to get up to the low forties, with sunshine at least until the afternoon. I called Marvin, who alerted the backhoe operator at the county garage and contacted County Sheriff Bobby Hammons. Later that morning, we all met at the graveyard.

The weather report had been a bit optimistic. The clouds were gray and lowering as we arrived at the cemetery, and the day was bitterly cold. Somehow, the bleak weather seemed appropriate for our morbid task—but I could have done without the sleet, which started to come down lightly, then heavily, after I'd been down in the grave for an hour or so.

"You going to be much longer, Doc?" Marvin called down after about five minutes of heavy sleet.

"Maybe another hour?" I called back. I was cold, too, but at least I was down here out of the wind—and moving. Poor Marvin and the sheriff had nothing to do but stand in the open cemetery and wait for us to hand up more bones.

·   ·   ·

When we finally got the bones back to the lab, I was eager to do my own analysis. Marvin had been right about one thing: Forensic science had advanced a good deal in the last thirty years, and I was sure I could find out more than my predecessors had. Although the people who had done the analysis thirty years ago had been expert pathologists, they didn't have the benefit of modern forensic techniques or of anthropologic expertise. And this victim's soft tissue had been badly decomposed when they found her, making it even harder to base an age estimate upon pathological evidence. As an anthropologist, I was trained to pick up on things that the previous scientists might have missed.

One thing I saw right away was that the woman was much older than they had thought. By my estimation, she was in her mid-twenties instead of in her teens—another indication that she might be Bobbie Taylor.

When I had finished a standard analysis of the bones, I sent the DNA sample down to LabCorp, the private DNA laboratory in North Carolina that would later analyze the genetic material of Henry Scharf.

Then, all we could do was wait. Two months later, on April 28, 1998, the DNA testing comparing Tent Girl's genetic material with a sample from her sister confirmed what Todd had suspected from the first: Tent Girl and Barbara Ann Hackmann Taylor were one and the same.

When the Taylor family learned of the positive identification, they decided to return to Georgetown for the burial service they hadn't been able to have thirty years before. Because our community had more or less adopted Tent Girl, the entire extended family, including Bobbie's adult daughter, decided to leave her here, her monument intact, although they did add a simple plaque with her real name. Bobbie's husband was dead by then, and there was no chance for a trial to bring justice for Bobbie, but at least her family could come together for a last farewell.

It seemed as if everybody in Georgetown came to the service, trying to look at the family—and Todd—without seeming to stare. Todd, of course, was the hero of the day, with Rosemary, Bobbie's daughter, and the rest of the family clustered around him, thanking him again and again for not giving up on his quixotic quest. I wished we could have told the family who killed Bobbie and promised them some kind of justice for her lonely death. But as I watched Rosemary and her niece shaking Todd's hand and patting him on the back, tears of relief streaming down their faces, I was glad that at least we had been able to give Tent Girl back her rightful name.

•　　•　　•

The story of Tent Girl evokes for me one of the most important—and poignant—parts of my job: victim identification. It's the police's job to catch the killers. It's my job to analyze the remains, which often starts and ends with figuring out who the person was, so that the law enforcement team—or the family—can take it from there. Much as I like working with the investigators, it's important for me to remember that their job is fundamentally different from mine. And if I forget that basic difference, I might get into real trouble when it comes time to testify in court. It's important for all parties—the lawyers for both sides, the judge, and above all the jury—to see me as supremely neutral, simply there to tell the scientific truth as I see it. If I ever once seem to be part of the prosecution's team—if I ever start to think of myself that way—my value to the process will be lost.

Because so much of crime drama and detective fiction focuses on catching the bad guys, my part of the process comes in for a lot of misrepresentation. In addition to everything else, movies, TV, and mystery novels often make my job seem a lot simpler than it is. If you don't know any better, you might get the idea that there's some kind of national database out there, recording every detail about every missing person in the country. You might easily come to believe that once the police have found an unidentified body, that magical computer will spit out an instant match.

Nothing could be further from the truth. Hundreds of people go missing every day—and, for many, nobody even bothers to report their absence. Say a family has a troubled teen at home, perhaps even a child who is being abused. The child runs away and the family—angry or ashamed or simply confused—doesn't report it. If that youngster's body turns up three states away with no identification, how can investigators ever give it a name? People don't come with bar codes. If someone asks us to compare a set of bones to the medical or dental records of Mary Smith or José Lopez, that we can do. But to pull a name out of thin air—no.

Even when there are missing persons reports, matching them to a body or a set of remains can be tricky. There *is* a national database, the National Crime Information Center (NCIC), which theoretically serves as a clearinghouse for matching missing persons reports with reports of unidentified remains. However, valuable though it is, the NCIC has a number of limitations.

First, as I said, many missing persons simply don't show up in the database. Maybe their loved ones never thought to file a report—perhaps because they fear the police, or are living in denial, or are simply ashamed to admit that their husband, wife, or child has seemingly left without a trace.

Then, too, a missing persons report is not always a high priority for an overworked police department that might have more than its share of homicides, robberies, and assaults to deal with. Many departments wait till the end of each week to file their missing persons reports, or maybe even the end of each month. If I've got a set of remains in my lab, I might not find the matching report the first time I look—or maybe even the second. Of course, the loved ones might take weeks, months, or even years to go to the police in the first place. And let's not forget human error—some agencies simply neglect to put their reports in the database.

Then there are problems with the way the NCIC records forensic information. The database was originally designed to match up stolen property and fingerprints, and the original fingerprint system has been taken over by an automated fingerprint identification system (AFIS). NCIC is still the only code-based data system available to those of us who try to identify the dead. So if everyone collects all necessary data from both sides of the equation (missing on one side, unidentified on the other) and if there are enough correctly coded *unique* identifiers (dental records, tattoos, previously broken bones, etc.), investigators stand a good chance of finding a match—if there is one.

However, a great deal of biological information is simply subjective, and it may not show up in the objective language of computer matching. What if the missing person's report describes a daughter's hair as golden blond—and the investigator who finds the remains thinks of her hair as closer to red? Even if both reports are on file, the NCIC isn't going to match them up. The same goes for descriptions of tattoos or scars or any other distinguishing feature—it's hard to do a computer match by verbal description alone.

Missing persons reports are also legendary in their shortcomings because people don't necessarily know what kind of information will help investigators identify their loved ones. Most people's impulse is to describe a missing person as if they wanted to pick him or her out of a crowd—blond hair, blue eyes, mole on the left cheek. That's not necessarily the information that will help us make a forensic identification. Did she suffer from scoliosis when she was young? Does he have a broken bone that eventually healed, or has he maybe had some back surgery? Does she file her nails into a particular shape or use a unique polish? Is he a heavy smoker—enough to stain his teeth? Did she wear braces as a child? Do you even have his dental records or her medical records? Then, too, the people who take down missing persons reports aren't scientists and they don't necessarily know the kind of information we need.

In the end, the biggest difficulty in identifying missing persons is probably the sheer volume of people who seem to have simply vanished. The NCIC database contains literally hundreds of thousands of names, and for any search you conduct, you might easily get dozens, hundreds, or even thousands of matches. Trying to sort through every single one of these can be an investigator's nightmare.

Suppose, for example, that you find a set of bones in the woods that you identify as belonging to a middle-aged White man about six feet tall, of average weight, with no unique dental features, and with no unusual fractures, scars, or tattoos. Your best guess puts his age at thirty to forty, though you realize that you might be off by three or four years either way. You can only estimate how long he's been there or when he disappeared. If you put information like that into the NCIC database, you'd end up with probably a thousand matches, going back for at least ten years and extending over all fifty states and Canada.

Maybe you can narrow it down a bit. Perhaps your remains show evidence of a broken collarbone that healed shortly before death. So you ask to see only missing persons reports that mention such an injury. That should knock out lots of matches—but what if the person who filed the report didn't know about the collarbone or didn't bother to tell the police about it? Then there's no chance of a match even if your guy's report is in the system.

Or suppose you put the man's age at thirty to forty and he's actually forty-one? Your computer search will blithely eliminate the one report you need—while providing you with hundreds, maybe thousands, of reports that you don't need. (I always add an extra five years on either end of my age estimates for this very reason—even though it doubles, triples, or even quadruples the number of reports I have to sift through.)

I could go on and on. Women whose families add two inches to their height because they're used to seeing their loved one in high heels. Parents who give the police detailed descriptions of a son's tattoo—but the remains you're looking at were destroyed by fire or decomposed in a lake or have become totally skeletonized by the time you find them. The gaps between missing persons reports and unidentified remains are one of the most frustrating and heartbreaking parts of this job.

We've had some major breakthroughs in the last few years. The Internet is at the heart of most of these, and the new publicly available databases for missing adults are a tremendous help. Before these online services, only missing children had a national clearinghouse, through the National Center for Missing and Exploited Children. Now, with the help of the Internet, people whose adult loved ones are missing can be certain that the information on their parents, children, spouses, or friends will have a chance to go beyond the police department and out to the ordinary citizens who might be able to provide information.

Of course, sometimes you just get lucky. Or a flash of intuition mysteriously cuts through the statistics, as it did with Tent Girl. Sometimes, too, the Internet can be the vehicle for both luck and intuition, enabling identifications that can seem downright miraculous. Such was the case of Letitia Luna, a young woman who disappeared—seemingly into oblivion—on August 7, 2000.

·   ·   ·

For me, Luna's story began on August 14, 2000, when a Mississippi riverman discovered a waterlogged body caught between two barges traveling upstream to the Ohio River. The autopsy findings revealed that the remains had once been a White female, twenty to twenty-five years old, with long black hair and a slender build, clothed in jeans and a T-shirt. She also had a watch on her wrist and a pair of eyeglasses in her pocket. Although the body was badly decomposed, the medical examiner could still make out the faint traces of a rose tattooed on her wrist.

The Carlisle County coroner and the state police publicized the case along the western border of the state. Thinking that the woman had fallen or been thrown into the river and had then floated downstream, the police asked their colleagues in all of the river cities above them if they had a missing person who fit this description. They didn't.

About six months later, I got a call from Kentucky Medical Examiner Dr. Mark LeVaughn. Although Jane Doe's body was badly decomposed, there was still enough soft tissue left for a conventional autopsy, so no one needed me to analyze her bones. Instead, I was being called for my skills as a forensic artist: Mark thought I might be able to do a facial "restoration," a sketch based on autopsy pictures and forensic information.

"I'll give it a try," I offered, and asked to see the autopsy photographs. Ideally, I could use these as a template to create a sketch showing what the victim might have looked like when she was alive. Then the police would circulate the sketch widely, hoping that someone would recognize the person and come forward.

But when Mark sent me the photos, I realized they'd be no help. This young woman's face was far too decomposed for me to be able to draw a recognizable image of her.

The only other option was to boil her head in my Crock-Pot and use the clean, dry skull for a clay facial reconstruction. This was a time-consuming, chancy process—even with the best clay reconstruction or a good sketch, there was no guarantee that the right person would see it and come forward—so I wanted to exhaust all other chances of giving her a name. Since there was so much identifiable evidence associated with this victim, I persuaded the police and coroner to continue searching for her identity, promising to do a clay reconstruction—but only as a last resort.

Almost five months later, the young woman still didn't have a name, and I was scheduled to start the facial reconstruction on the following Monday. Now it was three o'clock on Friday afternoon, and I found myself in the unusual position of being done for the week. Acting on the same elusive intuition that had apparently driven Todd Matthews, I flipped on my computer and began yet another search of missing persons sites on the Internet. This was hardly the first time I'd done such a search—but, today, for some reason, I was drawn to the website operated by the Nation's Missing Children Organization and Center for Missing Adults (NMCO). Sometimes my eyes and brain make a mysterious connection that puts me into an almost trancelike state, and it was in this condition of heightened awareness that I flipped through the pictures in the missing persons gallery, one image at a time.

Suddenly, I stopped short. One of the pictures had seized my attention with a surprising force. There was no description with the photograph, but as I looked at the young woman—her shy smile, her long black hair—somehow, I just *knew*. This was the woman we'd been looking for.

The photo had a link to the detailed information that family members had supplied to the website, and I clicked on it immediately. Yes, everything was right—her age, her height, the time since death, her long black hair, even the rose tattooed on her wrist. And, I read eagerly, the young woman's car had been found on the DeSoto Bridge in Memphis—still running—about five hundred miles downstream from where our body was found.

Wait a minute—her car was found *downstream*? So her body had floated *upstream,* hundreds of miles against the Mississippi's mighty current? It hardly seemed possible. Unless somebody had taken her upstream, of course.

I didn't care. I knew our Jane Doe was Letitia Luna. Now all I had to do was prove it.

I called the Memphis police station, where a helpful detective gave me the name and phone number of Luna's dentist. As I waited for him to fax me her records, I called the detective back and she agreed to get in touch with Luna's family and obtain a detailed description of her tattoo. Then I called Mark LeVaughn and the Carlisle County coroner and offered up my tentative identification.

Back in Memphis, the detective I'd spoken to was searching the station's missing persons chart to see if there was any more information that we could use. She found a note affirming that Letitia had owned a pair of wire-rim glasses which she normally carried in her pocket, just as our Jane Doe had done.

It was now almost nine o'clock on a Friday evening, but with victory so close, I couldn't quit. I arranged for the Memphis detective to contact the family, and that night, Mark, Luna's dentist, Luna's family, and I e-mailed the dental records back and forth, along with pictures of the tattoo and the glasses. By ten a.m. Saturday, we had determined that everything did indeed match. The search for Letitia Luna was over.

•   •   •

I was enormously grateful to have Luna's dental records, because we'd had nothing else to secure a positive ID. The eyeglasses helped corroborate my hunch, but you can never base an ID on personal effects—there are just too many ways that someone might end up with another person's stuff: theft; a simple loan; a murderer's deliberate attempt to throw off suspicion; or the fiery confusion of a plane crash or exploding building, in which not only personal effects but also body parts become commingled.

So what can you use for a positive ID? Well, teeth are always good. As I'd told Marvin, you don't necessarily need the dental records—with a good photo and unusual teeth, you might be able to match the dental work in the photograph with some teeth in an actual skull. Dental records are nice, too, of course, though as I learned in the case of Henry Scharf, even dentists make mistakes.

You might be able to make a positive ID from a tattoo, if it's unusual enough and everything else fits. The rose on Luna's wrist wasn't unique, but both she and Jane Doe were also dark-haired, female, the same height, and missing about the same length of time. In Luna's case, I wouldn't have been willing to rely on the tattoo alone, because so many young women nowadays are tattooed, and small flowers, hearts, and butterflies are so common.

Fingerprints are also nice, though this type of evidence can be more subjective than most people think. You compare fingerprints by a system of points, and if you can't get enough points to match, you may not be able to make a positive ID. Of course, since I deal with bones and decomposed remains, the flesh from their fingertips is usually long gone or so badly decomposed that prints aren't possible.

Surgical hardware is another good basis for a positive ID. Since 1993, doctors have been required to record the individual serial number of many of the pieces of hardware they install in people's bodies, which certainly makes life easier for the folks in my office.

An x-ray might lead to a positive ID, if it reveals a sufficiently unusual body part—an ankle with a healed fracture, say, or a uniquely curved pair of finger bones. Or maybe someone has a strange growth on her elbow—something she never even knew she had—but it shows up on an x-ray in her antemortem medical file somewhere, a perfect match for your remains. Some bones, too, are as unique as fingerprints, such as the frontal sinuses—the air pockets in the forehead bone at the area right between and above the eyes. So if I'm lucky enough to have an antemortem x-ray showing a frontal view of the sinus area, I can compare that to John Doe's skull and get a positive ID out of that.

Of course, the ultimate positive ID is matching DNA. It's almost foolproof and it tends to put all questions to rest. However, it's only used as an absolute last resort. It's not like you can plug your Jane Doe's DNA into some big database—most people's genetic material is not on file. If you have some idea who your victim might be, you can ask his or her family for a matching sample. But if all you've got is dry bones, you have to match mitochondrial DNA. This is an expensive and

time-consuming method of identification. As of this writing, mitochondrial DNA extraction and comparison costs an average of five
thousand dollars and usually takes weeks or even months.

Sometimes you don't even get to the stage of a positive ID—the best
you can do is eliminate a bad choice. My office posts all our unidentified victims on a website, and every two weeks or so I get a call from
an investigator somewhere in the country, hoping to match his missing
persons report to my John or Jane Doe. We start checking through all
the variables: Okay, we can match the height, the weight, the time
since death. We might even find evidence of a striking tattoo or a broken arm that healed years ago.

Then he faxes me the dental records—and no dice. Our guy's teeth
may be similar, but they're not the same. We cross each other's names
off the list and go on to someone else.

For the process to work, of course, you need two kinds of reports
on file: missing persons and unidentified remains. When the Luna case
was over, I found myself wondering why the Memphis and Kentucky
police had never put their reports together.

The answer was simple—though profoundly embarrassing. For
some reason, although the Kentucky State Police had circulated details
about the case to local news outlets and police posts across the state,
they had never entered their information into the NCIC database. So
in addition to all the other factors that might make victim identification difficult, we have to add simple human error.

The Luna case also raises an interesting question about where to
look for a missing person. Before this case was solved, when you found
a body in a river, you tended to look upstream for its source, especially
if there was no evidence of foul play. But Luna's body had not been
shot or stabbed or strangled—she had obviously died by drowning—
and yet her body had come from downstream. Why?

The answer lies in the unique hydrology of the "duck ponds" created between two barges in a tow. The motion of the barges creates
eddy currents in these open spaces, sucking up the water and anything

else on or slightly below the surface, down to a depth of eighteen inches. Luna's body had somehow gotten caught in a duck-pond eddy and been pulled upstream with the barges. Now, my fellow investigators and I are all going back to other Jane and John Does that have been found in the Ohio River, looking downstream as well as upstream for missing persons reports they might match.

•   •   •

Of course, the toughest problem in identifying human remains is also the simplest: Where do you start? According to Kym Pasqualini, the founder and coordinator of the NMCO, the number of reported missing adults topped 43,000 in March 2003. When you add the number of missing children to the list, the total comes to a staggering 97,297.

Those numbers are daunting enough when you've got a victim with an unusual biological profile or a special piece of surgical hardware whose serial number might somehow be traced. But what about the thousands of victims who basically resemble thousands of others?

Such was the problem with the Jane Doe in Baraboo, Wisconsin, the one whose facial reconstruction I described in the prologue to this book. This was the young woman whose body parts had been butchered and flayed and carefully wrapped in grocery bags, which someone had then thrown into the Wisconsin River. Since months of searching for her by conventional means had failed, Sauk County Detective Joe Welsch and Wisconsin Special Agent Elizabeth Feagles had come to me, hoping I could do a facial reconstruction on her skull.

By the time I became involved with the case, forensic scientists in Wisconsin had already done a complete analysis of the remains, determining that the young woman so brutally butchered had been a young Black female, about twenty to twenty-five years old, probably about 5'2" and weighing 120–130 pounds. Wisconsin fingerprint expert Mike Riddle had even managed to lift prints from her decomposed hand— an almost superhuman feat that left me awestruck.

But all this science hadn't gotten them very far. According to the NCIC database, more than 1,500 women who fit that profile had been reported missing since early that summer. Getting the prints was terrific—but where could they find a match? Most people who aren't criminals don't have their fingerprints on file. If Joe and Liz had had any idea where to look, they could have tried to lift prints from one of the young woman's possessions. But until they had some idea of who their victim was, they were stuck.

Like so many other unidentified victims, the Baraboo Jane Doe was so frustratingly ordinary. Her teeth were perfect, with no restorations. She had no tattoos or scars and no evidence of previously broken bones. The D.A. hoped that her skull would hold some critical forensic evidence—some cut marks that might someday be matched to a weapon. That was why we were using the rapid prototyping technology to create a perfect replica of her skull. But so far the skull itself had yielded far too little information about this woman's identity.

When Liz and Joe came to me, I was their last resort. They hoped desperately that my facial reconstruction would give them a visual image that they could circulate throughout the state. If all went as we intended—and we all knew that it might not—someone would see the image I created, recognize the victim, and come forward.

So as I began my facial reconstruction that Labor Day weekend, I knew the stakes were frighteningly high. Until the police knew who Jane Doe was, they would never find her killer. If a serial killer was out there somewhere, we had given him virtual license to try again. If the killer were someone more ordinary—a boyfriend, spouse, relative, or friend—he might literally get away with murder, and a particularly brutal murder at that. There was one last chance to keep that from happening—and it was all up to me.

I tried to keep the image of this woman's mutilated flesh out of my mind and concentrate on the skeletal details. Although it was unusual to be starting with a laminated paper skull rather than one made of human bone, everything else about this reconstruction was perfectly ordinary—just like the victim. As always, I began by cutting tissue markers—small sections of rubber that mark the depth of tissue in various parts of the victim's face. I make my markers from the standard pink erasers that go into mechanical pencils—long thin tubes of rubber that I buy at the office supply store and cut to size with an ordinary X-Acto knife.

The length and positioning of these markers is based on standard anthropological formulas that tell me how deep the flesh is likely to be on a person's cheeks, forehead, chin, and elsewhere, based on his or her sex, race, and estimated weight. Carefully following these formulas, I glue close to two dozen markers at specific points all over the skull, in the middle of forehead, the bridge of the nose, the point of the chin, and other key places. Then I connect them with clay, using the bone structure as my guide.

The most tedious part of the job comes right at the beginning. Cutting the markers to the right length and placing each one in its precise position is a painstaking task made all the more stressful by my awareness that the slightest mistake might compromise the accuracy of my final result. Some of those little rubber cylinders are no more than an eighth of an inch long, so as I worked on the Baraboo case that Labor Day weekend, I needed a sharp knife and a steady hand. Soon, however, I became absorbed in the soothing—if somewhat boring—mechanics of cutting the twenty-three markers, numbering each one of them with a sharp pencil, and laying them all out in numerical order. After about an hour, I was ready to go back to the skull.

I'd already mounted the laminated prototype on a converted camera tripod, which I'd fitted with a big eyebolt that fit up inside the spinal cord opening known as the foramen magnum. My tripod has a large ball joint at its base, which allows me to rotate and tilt the skull until it is perfectly level, a position known as the Frankfurt horizontal. In this position, the eye sockets appear to be aimed straight ahead and I can draw an imaginary level line from the bottom of the eye orbit to the ear hole known as the external auditory meatus. I grabbed the small carpenter's level that I use for this task and centered it over the bottom of the prototype's eye orbits.

Then I reached for the mandible, which the Milwaukee team had also made out of laminated paper, and fit it into sockets located just in front of the ears, the temporomandibular joint. I fiddled with the paper jaw until it fit perfectly, opening and closing in a smooth gliding motion so that the teeth of the upper and lower jaw fit together in normal occlusion. I didn't want my statue gritting her teeth—she'd be harder to recognize that way—so I put a small plastic strut betwen her upper and lower teeth for that tiny bit of separation that creates a more natural look. Then I adjusted the mandible until I had created a slight bit of distance between it and the skull, to mimic the normal separation created by the articular cartilage and a small fibrous disk called a meniscus. I knew that each tiny detail might make the difference between a face that someone might recognize and one that looked just slightly "off."

If my Jane Doe had had unusual teeth, they might have helped someone recognize her, so I would have had her bare those striking teeth in a smile—a complicated procedure that would have required still more manipulation of the jaw, since when a person smiles, the jaw drops and pulls back a little. Then, when I added the clay, I'd have had to make the statue's nostrils flare a bit, crunch up the flesh under her eyes, and flatten the flesh across her upper teeth to almost nothing— subtle but crucial touches that could make a huge difference in the final product.

Luckily, I didn't have to do that here—this woman's mouth would be closed. The replica's teeth were perfectly shaped and placed, but they were coated with the same honey-brown resin that covered the rest of the skull, which would hardly give a natural look to the final result. Besides, there was nothing unusual about the woman's teeth, so once her mandible was seated correctly, I started gluing on the tissue markers.

Simply out of habit, I always start at the forehead, dipping the eraser into some all-purpose glue and holding it in place for a few minutes until the glue starts to set. It took me the rest of that afternoon to glue each marker onto the skull.

As the sun was beginning to set I started on the eyes. Each artist has his or her own method, but I tend to do the eyes as soon as possible, mainly because I don't like to see those empty sockets staring at me hour after hour after hour. It's also easier to adjust the eyes before I put on the clay.

Running my fingers lightly over the replica's eye sockets, I found the place where the palpable ligaments would be inserted—the tiny ligaments that anchor the corners of each eyelid. The insertion points are located by means of subtle bumps that I couldn't see, but that my fingertips found immediately. I marked each one with pen because that's where the corners of the eyelids would go, and I wanted to remain aware of that positioning through the rest of my work with the eyes.

If I'd been using an actual skull, I'd have put some cotton into the eye sockets to protect the fragile bones for further forensic analysis. On a replica, that wasn't an issue, but I did need to keep the eyes from falling backward into the sockets. Folded-up Kleenex worked quite nicely.

Then, using a small block of clay, I made a little pedestal for the first artificial eye, which I'd bought from a surgical supply house that makes eyes for people who need prosthetic implants. These false eyes look eerily realistic and come in all sorts of colors—for a Black woman, I had chosen the darkest brown available, with a slight yellow tinge to the surrounding "white" sclera. I stuck the eye onto its little clay pedestal and quickly mortared it into place with more strips of clay.

Soon both eyes were in and I began adjusting their position. I wanted my sculpture to have a perfect gaze—each eye centered precisely in its orbit, protruding just the right distance in relation to the surrounding bone. The eyes should be level, too, and they should look together in the same direction. One of my tricks is to shine a single bright desk lamp into the eyes and look at the reflection. In a perfect gaze, the light is reflected exactly the same way in both eyes, so I spent half an hour adjusting first one eye, then the other. My reward was a steady, earnest gaze resembling that of a living person.

I took a late dinner break and went back to apply the clay. Here was where my artistic intuition came into play. Although I am ultimately a scientist, I've learned over the years that simply following the mathematical formulas isn't enough. If my facial reconstruction is ever to come to life, I have to venture beyond the formula and allow my intuition to guide me to create all those individual little details that ultimately distinguish each face from every other. I have to make creative leaps—but leaps that are entirely supported by scientific data. It's this fusing of art and science that makes the difference between a scientifically correct but somehow vague face and a vivid, lively image that someone might actually recognize.

Luckily, my intuition had lots of data to work with. When Joe had brought me the skull, he'd also handed over several photographs taken at autopsy and a copy of the autopsy report. The pathologist had found that this young woman was basically healthy, with an average amount of well-distributed subcutaneous fat. Since her genitalia were still present, he'd known she was a female. He'd estimated her age based on the youthful condition of her internal organs—mature, but showing no age-related changes in the heart, reproductive organs, or arteries.

He had also determined that this woman was African American, based on the color of her very dark skin. Of course, skin color can undergo rapid and dramatic changes after death, but this woman had other Negroid features as well. The pathologist had mentioned her black, coarse, and extremely curly body hair. And despite the fact that her face was no longer visible—the flesh had literally been cut away from the bone—the anthropologic analysis of her skull told us that she had once had wide-set eyes; a well-rounded or "bossed" forehead; and a wide flat nose. Until I finished applying the clay, I would have said "African American," too.

But when my sculpture was done, something in the facial contours caught my eye. Somehow, the extreme flatness of the mid-face and the almost vertical shape of her front teeth and jaws made hers look different from the other African-American skulls I'd seen. Certainly, this woman wasn't White. But I couldn't quite believe she was a Black American, either.

What other choices were there? I e-mailed my concerns to Dr. Leslie Eisenberg, a consultant to the pathologist who had done the autopsy and one of the foremost anthropologists in the country. For a time, Leslie considered my speculation that the woman might be one of the native Hmong tribespeople from the mountains of Vietnam who had relocated to Wisconsin as a result of the Vietnam War. The Hmong have dark skin, too, and relatively flat facial features, but unlike this woman's, their hair is usually straight.

Maybe Indonesian, I suggested, and Leslie politely considered that possibility, too. Eventually, we both concluded that this woman was Black—but the unusual combination of features continued to bother me.

At least my reconstruction was done. I took another look at her innocent young face and wondered if we would ever find out who she was—and who had killed her. But my work wasn't done yet. I wanted my finished product to look as much like a person as possible. A forensic sculpture will never be as accurate as a sculptured portrait or "bust" that has been made from a photograph or taken from life. Because I have only the shape of the skull to guide me, any reconstruction I create will be an approximation at best, a caricature at worst: an artificial face with enough similarities to the victim that it might trigger recognition in someone, but far from a perfect portrait. So I wanted to give all possible help to the man or woman who might see my work, to increase the chance that he or she would recognize our victim.

I placed a long black wig on the sculpture and combed it carefully into place. Later, I'd try out two or three other wigs, taking photographs of each version. Meanwhile, I "dressed" my statue in a pink striped T-shirt, and for an extra touch of realism I dabbed fresh lipstick over the lips, just enough to add a little color and shine.

I'd created the sculpture at home, but I arranged to meet Joe and Liz at my office before work that Tuesday morning, exhausted but excited after my three-day working weekend. Liz, I knew, had been skeptical from the beginning about Joe bringing in an outsider—a Kentucky artist to solve a Wisconsin case. Like most law enforcement investigators, she was a bit territorial, especially about such a high-profile case—and I later learned that she'd worked several other cases in which facial reconstructions had proved futile. Though she had little faith in this effort, Joe was eager but reserved, his eyes continually wandering to Liz to check out her reactions.

"Come on back to my lab," I said after the introductions were made. I pointed to my sculpture, sitting on the counter in the center of the room, and waited.

When they saw it, the expression on their faces didn't change and neither of them said a word. Each of them glanced quickly at me and then back at the model. Joe reached out to touch the hair, and Liz gently placed her hand on his wrist to stop him.

I was sure they hated it. Nervously, I broke the silence with a lengthy description of the digital photographs I had taken of my work, assuring them that the computer printouts minimized the little flaws and surface irregularities that showed up so glaringly in the clay. "You can see here—" I began, pointing to the pictures lined up on the counter beside the model. Liz shook her head and I fell silent again.

"And I've got these other wigs—" I began once more, reaching for them. This time Liz held up one palm for silence.

I searched desperately for my well-worn explanations of the limits of forensic sculpture. How it could never be portrait-quality—we just don't have the data for that. How, nevertheless, many people seem able to leap over the crude quality of a forensic image and jump to a flash of recognition, particularly when a loved one is involved. How often I had seen forensic images succeed—and, to be honest, how often I had seen them fail.

But to my utter surprise, the two of them began to smile and then to laugh.

"This is amazing," Joe said softly.

"More than amazing," Liz agreed. She turned to me. "I thought you'd do some kind of Gumby-like thing—I don't know, something that looked weird and unnatural. But this really looks like a human being. We might really find her with this."

. . . .

Three months later, nurse-practitioner Shari Goss saw the four photos of my facial reconstruction posted on the bulletin board of her neighborhood grocery store and burst into tears. "I know her," she told the astonished grocer. She had recognized Mwivano Mwambashi Kupaza, a young exchange student from Tanzania who had been living in Madison, Wisconsin, for the past three years. Kupaza was the twenty-five-year-old cousin of forty-year-old Peter Kupaza, Goss's ex-husband. After seeing the poster, Goss called the police in her rural Wisconsin hometown of Wesby to give them the young woman's name.

Joe and Liz were then able to find a photograph of Mwivano, which resembled my reconstruction almost exactly. They went on to match the prints lifted from the remains they had found with fingerprints lifted from medical records that Mwivano had touched when she signed them. Finally, we had our positive ID.

The story that Joe and Liz eventually put together was heartbreaking. They believed that Peter had raped Mwivano, who became pregnant and then had an abortion. About two years later, he allegedly killed her and dismembered her body in his home, packing it in plastic bags and carrying it to the river.

Ironically, no one had ever filed a missing persons report on Mwivano Kupaza. Her friends and relatives in Tanzania believed she was still in the United States. Her U.S. community of friends and fellow students thought she had returned to Tanzania.

Peter Kupaza's trial was a dramatic event. Mwivano's and Peter's relatives flew in from Tanzania, sitting in the front row for every day of the trial. When Shari Goss testified against her ex-husband, she nearly broke into tears as the D.A. showed her several knives that the couple had once had in their kitchen. Prosecutors suggested that these were the very knives that had been used to dismember Mwivano's remains. On another day, prosecutors showed a slow-motion video superimposition comparing my clay reconstruction to Mwivano's photograph.

There were audible gasps from the jury, and two of Mwivano's relatives began to cry.

Peter maintained his innocence throughout. A June 21, 2000, article by Jason Shepard in the *Capital Times* reported his testimony: "I would like to tell you today, I did not do this. I did not do this. I do not have the heart. . . . I miss my cousin." Shepard reported that Kupaza spoke of his and Mwivano's relatives as a single family. David and Rebecca Mwambashi were Mwivano's parents and Peter's aunt and uncle. Yet he spoke of them and of his uncle Raphael as though they were all his parents and as though Mwivano were his sister:

"Why should I make my father Raphael Mwambashi cry? Why should I make my father David Mwambashi cry? Why should I break his heart? . . . Why should I make my mother Rebecca cry forever? . . . Why should I do this to my sister? I'm supposed to protect her."

Yet Peter's own uncle, the family patriarch, Raphael Mwambashi, testified against his nephew. "He cheated me," Mwambashi was quoted as saying in the same article. "Now we know he was never true to me."

When Peter Kupaza was finally found guilty, he himself began to weep, while family members stared straight ahead, silently. Later, he was given a life sentence with no parole for thirty years—a decision that would mean he could not return to Tanzania until he was seventy years old. Although Mwivano's family had originally intended to take their daughter back with them, they decided to bury her remains in Wisconsin. Devout Lutherans, they chose to hold her funeral at Coon Prairie Lutheran Church in Westby.

"The burden is not as heavy as we thought it would be because of you people," Raphael Mwambashi said at the ceremony, according to a June 26, 2000, story by William R. Wineke in the *Wisconsin State Journal*. "We leave for home tomorrow having accomplished everything we had to do. We leave her body with you people knowing that it is in the good hands of good people." Although I could not be at the funeral, I was glad to have been part of the process that brought justice to the family of Mwivano Kupaza.

• • •

In the Kupaza case we had a skull, which helped enormously: It meant that we could give the victim a face, which enabled us to give her a name. But what if you don't have a skull? Some murderers know how useful those head bones are to crime scene investigators, and they go to no end of trouble to disguise the identity of their victims. Then we have to tease secrets out of something else.

Such was the case with Everett Hall, a disabled coal miner from Pike County, Kentucky, whose wife persuaded her two boyfriends to kill him in 1996. ("That woman had some awesome powers of persuasion," one of the deputies once told me.) Mrs. Hall's two beaux allegedly shot Everett in the head and decided to hide his body in a nearby abandoned coal mine, expecting his corpse to decompose rapidly. But when they went back to check on their work a year later, they discovered that the mine's consistent temperature, low humidity, and absence of flies and their larvae had simply mummified the remains. So they cut off Everett's head, burned it, and buried it in a construction site. To this day, that head reportedly lies beneath a small strip mall in Pikeville.

Now, thought the boyfriends, the head problem was solved—but what about the rest of the body? Hall's wife and her fellas decided to dynamite that section of the mine—but none of them had the cash to buy the dynamite. Hall's wife agreed to trade sexual favors for the explosives they needed—a maneuver that the detectives on the case would later dub "nookie for nitro."

The plan worked fine up until the actual explosion, when the guys failed to detonate the charge correctly. The disappointingly small blast only loosened a few small slabs of stone and filled the shaft with coal dust.

They decided to try again, since it would be years before enough coal dust settled to fully conceal the headless corpse. So they loaded Everett's remains into a wheelbarrow, rolled him into a more confined area of the mine shaft, and sent Mrs. Hall out for some more dynamite.

Unfortunately for them all, she only came back with a homemade hand grenade. Making do with what they had, the men rigged an elaborate system of pulleys and string to detonate the grenade after they were out of harm's way. But their second attempt was doomed to failure, too, for their weapon turned out to be nothing more than a smoke grenade.

After the smoke cleared, the men came up with a third plan. They decided to build a fire from the timbers that were holding up the roof of the mine, placed the corpse on their makeshift funeral pyre, and doused the whole thing with motor oil. Then, somehow, their survival instincts clicked into place. Realizing that they were in imminent danger of being crushed by a collapsing mine if not suffocated by the smoke filling a small, confined area, they decided not to light the fire and simply walked away, leaving the body still sprawled over the stacked timbers.

Despite the cartoon-like quality of these criminal efforts, Hall's murder was never discovered, and we might never have found the body if one of the men hadn't been arrested on an unrelated felony charge a year later. He gave up the story as part of some legal maneuvering, and I was called in when the detective who first entered the mine saw that parts of the body were skeletonized. Fearing that their own recovery of the remains might damage crucial evidence, local law enforcement officials asked me to take over.

I got the call late in the day, and I knew it would be almost dark by the time I drove over to Pike County, which is right on the West Virginia border. Still, it was going to be pitch dark in the mine at any hour, so this was one case where the time of day really didn't matter.

I'd never been inside a coal mine before, and the two-hour drive to the scene gave my imagination plenty of time to run wild. I seemed to recall every movie or television show I'd ever seen in which people got trapped inside a collapsing mine shaft or a secluded cave, leaving them without light or air—a fantasy that started to seem more and more real as the sun set and the sky grew darker.

My actual arrival on-site did nothing to calm the fears. As I was climbing into my jumpsuit and strapping on my kneepads, Pike County Coroner Charles Morris came up to me and said, "You know, Doc, you don't have to go in there if you don't want to. Those mine inspectors started talking after I called you up here, and although they assured me that the mine was safe, they were a little worried about sending in a woman who'd never been in a coal mine before."

I stared silently at him for at least five seconds while my mind raced. Everyone had turned to look at me and I knew I'd be judged by what I said next. I took a deep breath.

"First of all, Charles, nobody is *sending* me into that mine. I'm walking in *with* those guys who are telling you it's safe." I pointed directly at the men from the Bureau of Mine Safety and chuckled a little to soften my words, but I was serious as I added, "Of course, if they choose to stay out here in the open, I'll be right out here with them."

I could see the investigators nodding to each other, and that gave me the courage to go on. "Besides, Charles, how bad can it be? There's the entrance, and it's a lot bigger than I expected. Heck, it looks like it's eight feet high and a good fifteen feet wide. I've been in lots of spaces smaller than that."

This time it was the mine inspectors who laughed, and if I'd been a little more astute to the glances that passed between them, maybe I would have swallowed my pride and stayed outside. But I didn't. With my best show of bravado, I reached for my regular hard hat and picked up my biggest flashlight.

"No, Doc, that won't do," said Charles. "You have to wear this." He handed me a dented and blackened coal miner's helmet and a flat metal box to which was attached a short insulated cable and small spotlight. As I held this helmet in one hand and the box in the other, he strapped a thick nylon webbed belt around my waist.

"Put on the helmet first, Doc, and I'll adjust it for you."

I did as I was told. The headgear fit surprisingly well after Charles gave a little twist to a knob at the back of my neck, just under the helmet's rim. Next he took the flat orange-colored box from me and hooked it onto the belt.

"This here's the battery for that light you still have in your hand," he explained. "It's fully charged and should last as long as you're in there—unless, of course, you get lost or trapped." He looked me straight in the eye, but couldn't keep a straight face for long. I expect he spotted the apprehension that was starting to creep back into my eyes as I watched some of the mine inspectors shaking hands and wishing "good luck" to the folks who would be leading me inside.

"Hey, Doc, I was just kidding," Charles said in what I think he meant as a reassuring tone. He grabbed the cable attached to the battery and snaked it up through a loop in the back of my helmet, clipping it and the spotlight to the metal frame over my forehead. Then he clicked the light on and off a few times, just to make sure it worked. It gave off a bright white beam that seemed powerful enough in the dim twilight—but what kind of illumination would it provide once I was underground?

"Looks like you're good to go now, Doc," Charles said cheerfully. "Give me a minute to get my stuff on, and we'll join the others. Maybe you could grab that body bag and my camera from the back of that pickup over there while I suit up."

As we walked over to the mine entrance, Charles took the bag and the camera, leaving me free to walk into the mine with empty hands. As nonchalantly as I could, I turned on my light, pulled on my favorite leather gloves, and followed the other five members of the recovery team, who all finally turned on their own helmet lights and divided into pairs. We walked upright and side by side for about two hundred yards into the base of the mountain. By now, the last of the outside light had faded away and our tiny headlamps cast eerie shadows as they bounced along in cadence with our footsteps.

Then, suddenly, the shaft narrowed dramatically, like a funnel, the sides and ceiling closing in until there wasn't room to walk abreast or even to stand upright. That's when I noticed the silence. We were so far underground that no outside sound could penetrate, and I suddenly felt a wave of panic, gasping for breath and breaking out in a cold sweat.

"Wait up a minute, guys," I called to the men ahead of me. I had stopped dead in my tracks, trying to get control of my breathing. "I'm having a little trouble, here."

Newcomer's jitters were old hat to them, so they all stood together in a group, waiting for me to gather the courage to continue. I could tell they were amused by my discomfort, and more than one derisive glance was cast my way; but, frankly, I didn't care. I thought I was doing pretty damned good to have come *this* far!

Charles did, too. From this point on, he kept up a running commentary about the case, knowing that would keep my mind too busy to conjure up images of danger.

"We know who this guy is supposed to be, Doc. He disappeared about a year and a half ago, and the fella who told us where he hid the body said he helped with the killin'. While we were waiting for you to get here, I went ahead and collected a batch of the victim's x-rays, so hopefully you can identify him at tomorrow's autopsy. I think I told you that the head's been cut off, and it looks like maybe rats or something's been working on his fingers. There's no skin or prints left."

By now, I was stooped over and proceeding in a duck-walk crouch, a position so uncomfortable that it was hard to keep my mind on the case. My poor knees and back were about to give out, and my only comfort was that the situation couldn't possibly get any worse.

And then, of course, it did. Suddenly, the men in front of me stopped and one hung a lantern light on a hook that had been drilled into a single support timber.

"This is it," he said, pointing to a pile of jumbled coal and flat rocks. "From here on in, we'll be on hands and knees, but you've gotta be careful not to hit any of the support timbers on the other side of this pile. For some reason, the men who killed this guy pulled out most of the supports. I think the ones left are good enough to keep this shaft open, but this batch of rocks fell just as we were coming in to look for the body this morning, so let's not take any chances."

You don't have to worry about me, I thought. I had taken all the chances I was going to take just by coming down here in the first place.

Apparently without fear, the leaders of our team lay down and slithered through an opening that was just high enough to accommodate the bulk of an average-sized man. Swallowing hard, I followed them. After crawling a seemingly endless hundred yards on our hands and knees, we rounded a sharp corner and entered a slightly larger cavern about a mile and a half inside the mine, where Everett Hall had lain for the past eighteen months. His mummified corpse was perched on its belly on top of a pile of mine timbers, pointing a bony finger straight at us.

The space we had to work in was a little larger but no higher than the shaft we had just crawled through, allowing just enough room for my five helpers to sit down with their backs against the wall. Here they sat, aiming their headlamps at the corpse, waiting for me to make the next move.

This was my chance to make up for that panic attack, so I crawled casually over to the corpse and started dictating into my tape recorder.

The headless body is prone and is lying on top of a pile of wood. The body appears to be mummified from prolonged exposure to an environment with constant temperature and low humidity. There is no evidence of insect or maggot activity, but there is evidence of carnivore scavenging. The flesh has been removed from the torso and arms, and small tooth marks are visible in the remaining soft tissues. The lower portion of the body is wrapped in a dark-colored sleeping bag, and several pieces of rope and electrical wire encircle the sleeping bag. The body appears to be covered in a dark, unidentified viscous liquid . . .

"What is this stuff?" I said, interrupting myself. I held my fingers up to my nose trying to get a whiff of the greasy liquid. "It smells like my old car."

"It's gotta be either motor oil or kerosene," said Charles as he lifted a plastic jug from somewhere behind the corpse. "There's four of these jugs back here, and they're all empty. No miner in his right mind would bring this stuff in here, so these fools must have planned to burn this body on top of what looks like a makeshift bonfire."

"So it's flammable?" the rescue team leader jumped in, a hint of alarm in his normally easygoing voice. "All right, people, let's be extra careful. No camera flashes, and no scraping with these tools we brought. All we need is for a spark to reach this stuff, and we're all dead."

Okay, but what's the *good* news, I found myself thinking. I had never wanted to leave a crime scene so badly in my life. I picked up the few stray finger bones that had fallen to the floor of the mine and tried to think how to get the body out of this tight spot without causing any further damage to it. But scared as I felt, I had a job to do. Someone had to take pictures of the body before I moved it—and without a flash.

I glanced over at the four men sitting against the wall, their arms and legs folded like a row of Buddha effigies, and got an idea. "I know you guys don't want to get too close to this body, but I need you to scoot over here and give Charles and me some light. If you all aim your headlamps at one section at a time, I think there will be enough light to take some photos."

Praise the Lord, my idea worked, and soon we were ready to move the body. But now there was a new problem: The corpse had hardened and warped over time, so that parts of it were wedged between the pile of wood and the roof of the mine. With little room to maneuver in the confined space, I lay on my back and pushed up against the mummified torso from below, so that Charles could quickly slide out some of the heavy mine timber that had been supporting the victim's shoulders. Then I had to slide over and do the same thing to the lower legs, which were still wrapped in the sleeping bag. Somehow we managed to slide the body into the body bag that Charles had laid out on the floor of the mine.

Now Charles took over. "Okay, men. The doc here has done her part. Now we need you to help us get this fellow out of here."

I took a secret pleasure in seeing that everyone else was as eager as I was to leave, springing into action before Charles had even finished speaking. Luckily, someone had thought to bring some rope, which they tied into two loops at the end of the body bag in order to drag it through the shaft. Since there wasn't enough room to stand up and carry it, each man took turns slowly dragging it behind him as we crawled out of the shaft. When we reached the place where we could stand up again, our pace quickened as four men each grabbed a corner of the bag and carried it the rest of the way.

I breathed a sigh of relief when we got outside, silently vowing that I would *never* go into another coal mine. If there was another body down there, the mine inspectors or the coroner could bring it out *to* me.

.   .   .

Getting the body out of the mine felt like a huge achievement, but we still had to establish a positive ID, even though the state police and the coroner were sure that this was Everett Hall. I felt pretty confident, though, especially since Charles had brought a half-inch-thick stack of x-rays over to my lab in Frankfort. With all that medical data, it seemed pretty certain that we could quickly confirm his identity.

At first everything went smoothly. The pathologist conducted an autopsy that revealed a match between our victim's remains and the description on Everett Hall's missing person report, including the presence of a partially amputated foot that had healed quite nicely. Then it was my turn. I wheeled the gurney into the radiology room. I was fairly certain that once I took my first x-ray of the victim's spine, I'd be able to match my work to the films in Hall's medical records. I went to stand behind the lead-lined protective barriers in our lab's x-ray suite—built to hospital specification—and took my first shot.

It didn't match.

Okay, maybe I'd just gotten the angle wrong. I took another look at the films in the medical records, readjusted the body, and tried again.

Again, it didn't match.

I kept taking shot after shot until, I had taken more than ten x-rays of the victim's spine. No matter how I tried, I couldn't get a match.

When you're looking at antemortem spinal x-rays, you always start with the most current ones, because vertebrae tend to change shape slightly over the years, under the pressures of stress and advancing age. As time goes by, small overgrowths of bone called "lipping" commonly occur around the edges of each back bone. In this case, the x-rays in Hall's medical file showed significant lipping and partial collapse of one vertebra, but our victim had neither. Sometimes a person gets surgery to correct such problems, but there was no evidence that Hall had done that.

Was it possible that we didn't have Hall after all? Then why had this body appeared in exactly the same spot, under the same bizarre conditions, that had been described by Mrs. Hall's boyfriend?

Maybe the hospital had mislabeled these last few x-rays and put them in the wrong jacket? But when I looked carefully at the many x-rays in the envelope, every single one had the same name and patient number, affixed at the time of each x-ray exam. For three days, I tried to come up with a logical explanation for the discrepancy, while the authorities back in Pikeville grew increasingly impatient for the positive ID that would enable them to arrest their suspects and charge them with the murder of Everett Hall. In frustration, I went to Dr. Tracey Corey, one of the pathologists in our Louisville office, who thought a bit and then asked me whether Hall had been on Medicaid. When I told her that he was, she suggested that I compare all the x-rays in his file to one another.

Sure enough, they didn't match. It seemed that Hall's file contained the x-rays of three separate people—all listed under the same name and patient identification number. Apparently, Hall had been passing around his Medicaid card to others who also reaped the benefits of free medical care at taxpayers' expense. I had to go back through the entire file, all the way to 1986, to find some x-rays that actually matched our victim's spine.

I learned a valuable lesson from Hall's case, because I have since

encountered three similar cases of medical fraud while trying to identify homicide victims from x-ray comparisons. I guess when you're trying to establish a positive ID, you can never be too careful.

·   ·   ·

Sometimes the evidence you need for a victim ID has been destroyed,
either by accident or by the deliberate efforts of a murderer. In a case
I later thought of as "Ashes to Ashes," I had to go to extraordinary
lengths to recover human remains from fire-related debris—a painstaking process, but one that paid off in the end.

Gary and Sophie Stephens were a well-respected and popular couple who lived in the Coldiron community in Kentucky's Harlan
County. They vanished shortly after an evening church service in
December 1997. Although their son, a U.S. postal worker, lived with
them, he claimed to have no knowledge of their whereabouts.

Authorities duly got a search warrant and examined the house,
where they found minute traces of blood spatter and a single bullet hole
in the wall. An all-out effort by the community sent searchers into the
mountains, forests, and coal mines throughout the county for a nonstop three-day search.

Finally, a neighbor found the Stephenses' abandoned pickup truck
behind a tobacco barn. Detectives had it loaded onto a flatbed truck and
taken to a commercial garage, where they went over the truck with a
fine-tooth comb. When they found what appeared to be fragments of
burned bone behind the toolbox, they called me.

A two-hour drive got me to the garage in Loyall where they had
delivered the truck. No one answered my knock on the door, but after
I blew the horn of my van a few times, the garage door opened and
several state troopers signaled for me to drive right inside. No wonder
they hadn't heard me knock—a long cylindrical kerosene heater was
roaring in the center of the room, and the guys had a radio blaring to
try to drown out the noise. The sound was not pleasant, but the

warmth certainly was. It was now seven p.m. and already well below freezing.

"Glad you got here so quick," said a detective I knew only as Smitty. "Philip's out by the river, but he'll be back in a few minutes."

I had never worked a case in Harlan County, but I knew Coroner Philip Bianchi from some of the classes I had taught for coroners in the Commonwealth, and I recognized most of the officers from having worked dozens of cases in the surrounding region. After the obligatory handshakes all around, Smitty helped me out of my coat and directed me to a pickup covered with a blue tarp.

"Philip asked if you would go ahead and look at the stuff in the truck as soon as you got here. We need to make sure these are human bones."

Indeed they were—incinerated human bone fragments mixed in with the ashes and dirt that had sifted into the corners of the truck bed. I had the impression that the truck bed had been swept out, but not completely, leaving these bits and pieces behind.

When Smitty heard that these fragments were human, he picked up his radio to call the coroner and the other investigators, who had been searching the area for two bodies. But neighbors had already told troopers about seeing the Stephens boy near a large blaze in the woods that had apparently been burning for about two days. Though fires are common in rural Kentucky to clear fields and destroy garbage, it was starting to look like this particular bonfire might have been Gary and Sophie's final resting place.

It was already dark out, and a bitter wind was blowing. But troopers headed out to the site of the bonfire, surrounded the scene with crime scene tape, and blocked the road. Some of the men fanned out to talk with local residents, who told them that the Stephenses' pickup had also been spotted along a railroad track that ran parallel to the Cumberland River, a few miles out of town at a place called Big Rock. A trooper drove over there, then hiked down the path leading to the huge rock that jutted out over the river. As her flashlight played over the craggy landscape, she could see ashes and bones on the rocks that led down to the shore, some just inches away from the water. She quickly put up more crime scene tape by the railroad tracks and radioed Smitty.

Back at the garage, we were all monitoring the radio and making plans for tomorrow. We'd have to process at least three crime scenes— the truck, the bonfire, and the rocks by the river.

"Let's start with the easy one," I told Smitty. We could do the truck tonight, in fluorescent light and relative warmth. I felt sorry for the troopers who would have to babysit the other two crime scenes all night, but I was soon absorbed in the challenge of getting bone fragments out of the truck.

It wasn't easy. The tiny shards were so badly burned that they often crumbled and slipped through my fingers. Things went a little better when I figured out that I could use a hand trowel, slipping the tool gently under the ashes and laying them on a bed of folded toilet paper that lined the bottom of one of my plastic boxes.

I cleared out the truck bed, but that was only part of the job. Bone fragments and ashes had sifted back behind the toolbox, under the hinges of the tailgate, and behind the bumper where we couldn't reach.

Of course, I could rinse the truck out with a water hose, but what would happen to the skeletal evidence? If I was ever going to identify the victims, I'd need every piece of bone or tooth that remained. It was already touch and go whether we'd find anything that could be compared to Gary and Sophie's medical and dental records. I couldn't bear to think of a critical piece of evidence being washed down the drain.

When I finally figured out a solution, Smitty and the others laughed, but they agreed to help me out. We rolled the truck over to a large drain in the floor of the garage and used a couple of car jacks to tip the truck sideways and backward, so that the rear left corner of the truck bed was lower than the rest. Then we fitted one of my small-mesh sifting screens over the drain and began hosing out the truck as gently as we could.

By midnight, we had enough particles to fill a two-gallon bucket. I covered the bucket in heavy plastic sealed with some duct tape, so I could examine it more closely when I got back to the lab.

Philip had arranged for me to spend the rest of the night in a local motel, and I was grateful for a nice warm bed. My van is always packed and ready to go, with a toothbrush, clean clothes, and a dry pair of boots there when I need them. And boy, did I need them this time!

I worked side by side with Philip and the state police for the next two days, in subzero temperatures, collecting bones and tooth fragments from six different sites. The killer had tried hard to eliminate the remains, but fire is rarely as thorough as we think. There's almost always some part of the body left behind, though sometimes it can be hard to spot.

At the bonfire, for example, we found human bone fragments and blood, evidence that at least one of the victims had been incinerated here. An arson investigator determined that the ground had been soaked with kerosene and scoured with a rake, the killer stirring the fire until only fragments and ashes remained. The killer had then apparently loaded the remaining rubble into the bed of the pickup truck and driven it out of the woods, but bumps along the way shook loose some of the evidence, so we also found a small pile of ash containing human bone fragments on that rocky dirt road. As my colleagues and I carefully followed the trail of ash, collecting and documenting it as we went, I couldn't help thinking of the little birds that had picked up Hansel and Gretel's trail of bread crumbs.

We found another pile of bone-filled ash at the head of the path leading to Big Rock, as well as tracks that matched the tires on the Stephenses' pickup truck. The path bordered on a steep cliff that fell almost straight down into the Cumberland River, whose swift icy waters had undermined the limestone and created a large, swift pool that was more than ten feet deep and swirled with several large whirlpools. I imagined that the killer had stood at the edge of Big Rock and thrown most of the ash into the river, but clumps of bone and ash still clung tenaciously to rocks at the water's edge.

That let me in for a harrowing two days of rappeling to the water's edge, balancing on ice-covered rocks as I used a paintbrush to ease human ash out of the crevices and into a dustpan, then transferred all of it to plastic boxes lined with a cushion of toilet paper. Meanwhile, the police brought in a team of scuba divers from Louisville to check out the river bottom, where they recovered a few more bone fragments.

Back at the lab, I was faced with the daunting task of sifting through some eighty pounds of ash mixed with dirt and fire debris. All of us knew who these victims were—but I was the one who had to prove it, hopefully while finding enough evidence to allow the medical examiner to confirm a cause and manner of death.

By this point, I knew that the largest and most revealing pieces of bone had been recovered from the riverbank, so I opened those boxes first, carefully lifting out the forty-three bone fragments, one by one, onto a clean white sheet of butcher paper. When I saw two complete femoral heads, each from the top end of a right thighbone, I knew we had the remains of two people. But I couldn't yet prove who they were. Philip had found Gary and Sophie's medical and dental records, but I hadn't yet found any teeth or bone fragments that I could match to them.

The sorting process was slow and tedious, but I figured out how x-rays might help. I transferred scoops of ash onto a fiberglass cafeteria-style tray, gently smoothing the debris with my fingertips until it was only an inch thick. Then I took an x-ray of the tray, looking at the films to spot the difference between bone, wood, and metal. When I spotted something that piqued my interest, I could lay the x-ray film right on top of the tray, pinpointing the location of the exact piece I wanted.

I sifted my way through hundreds of scoops of ash, picking out several large pieces of bone, teeth, and metal chunks. Then, after about twelve hours of this sorting process, I saw something that made my heart stop. There on an x-ray was a U-shaped piece of metal with serrated edges. From my former career in orthopedics, I knew I had come upon a surgical fixation staple, most often used to repair or reconstruct ligaments in the knee. I found it hidden in the tray full of ash and rinsed it off well enough to see the engraved logo of the manufacturer and the model number.

I sprinted from the lab to my office, reaching for the pile of medical records stacked up on my desk. I searched desperately for proof of knee surgery—and there it was. Gary Stephens had undergone knee ligament repair in Knoxville just a few years earlier. A quick call to his doctor confirmed that the staple used in the operation was the exact same make, model, and size as the one I'd found.

One positive ID down and one to go. With a fresh wave of enthusiasm, I continued to x-ray several dozen more trays of debris, hoping to identify Sophie. It was a slow, unrewarding process as the x-rays turned up a discouraging number of dead ends—bits of metal that turned out to be zipper teeth, jean rivets, and even a couple of bootlace hooks.

True, I'd also recovered several small pellets of bird shot. But it's not that unusual to find loose shotgun pellets or even bullets in the homes, vehicles, or pockets of Kentucky's rural residents, so the shot was hardly proof of murder.

Then I did see something useful: a pellet of bird shot actually embedded in a fragment of bone from the spine. Holding my breath, I delicately flicked away the surrounding ash and smiled triumphantly. I now had proof that at least one of the victims had been shot.

There was still no proof that any of these ashes had once been Sophie's, however. And by noon of the third day, I was starting to lose hope. The only evidence that remained was the bucket of debris that we'd rinsed out of the pickup truck, and I'd already looked at that the first night, as it was dripping onto the screen. I hadn't seen anything important then and I didn't expect to find anything now.

Of course, now I had the advantage of x-ray vision. So I continued with my routine of scooping the ash, spreading it out, and scanning the x-rays. Hours passed without results. Then, as I was processing the very last handful of ash, I saw a strange silhouette—like nothing I'd seen in the previous three dozen x-rays. After I'd placed the film on top of the tray and filtered carefully through the mess, my fingertips seized on a small hard object. It was black and covered with ash, and I didn't recognize it until I rinsed it off in the sink. Then I breathed a final sigh of relief. There in my hand was the porcelain crown of a tooth—the very crown I could see on Sophie's dental records.

Now both victims had been identified and we could also prove that at least one of them had been shot in the back. The arson specialist could testify that someone had intentionally incinerated human bodies in the woods and I could attest that the ashes of two people had been thrown into the river. One of these was Gary Stephens. I could also prove that human bones and teeth had been found in the Stephenses' pickup truck, and that one tooth fragment belonged to Sophie.

Though it was impossible to completely separate the remains, it seemed appropriate to bury the husband and wife together, intermingled in death as they had been bound in life. When their son Gary was charged with their murders, he insisted on his innocence, but after he was faced with an impending death penalty trial in the autumn of 2002, he finally pled guilty and was sentenced to life imprisonment.

The "Ashes to Ashes" case taught me a valuable lesson—no detail is too small to be useful, especially when you're dealing with victims who have been destroyed by fire. Like the other cases in this chapter, it points out the many difficulties faced by those of us who try to identify human remains. These cases are hard enough when you are dealing with one victim at a time. When you throw in an explosion, a huge fire, and several dozen victims—the standard recipe for any mass fatality—identifying individuals becomes even more of a challenge. Yet, whether you're dealing with one victim or several hundred, the rules remain the same: Go slow, keep an eye out for details—and always be prepared to be surprised.

7

Oklahoma City

When will our consciences grow so tender
that we will act to prevent human misery rather than avenge it?
— ELEANOR ROOSEVELT

THE PLANE WAS JUST COMING in for a landing as I stuffed the academic journals into my briefcase. I'd already gone over them a hundred times back in Kentucky—after all, I myself had written ten several of these articles, and since I'd gotten the call from the FBI two days before, I'd reviewed them again and again—but I wanted to be sure I knew this material backward and forward. The FBI had called me in as a consultant on one of the largest law enforcement investigations in U.S. history—the bombing of the Murrah Federal Building in Oklahoma City—and I was taking no chances on not knowing my stuff.

It was August 31, 1995, and the FBI investigation into the bombing had been going on for four and a half months now. Danny Greathouse, the special agent in charge of the FBI's Disaster Identification Unit, had called me when the investigation first began. There were plenty of forensic specialists available—the ones that the FBI usually consulted at the Armed Forces Institute of Pathology (AFIP) and the Smithsonian Institution, as well as the excellent staff at the Oklahoma City Medical Examiner's Office. However, because I'd already worked one sensitive case for the FBI, at Waco, Special Agent Greathouse wanted to be sure he had backup if he needed it.

The victim identification process had continued on without me and I didn't think I'd be involved in the case. Then, two days ago, Special Agent Greathouse had called again, telling me to expect a call from Dr. Douglas Ubelaker. This time they didn't just need backup—they needed *me*. A major point in the case turned on the racial identification of a single dismembered leg, and Dr. Ubelaker knew that I'd published one article and a large section of my doctoral dissertation on the racial characteristics of the intercondylar notch, a portion of the distal femur at the knee. By one of those odd coincidences that seem to happen so often in my life, the very discovery I'd made when I'd solved the puzzle in Dr. Bass's class was the exact piece of knowledge that was needed here.

FBI Special Agent Barry Black met me at the Will Rogers World Airport and whisked me straight to the medical examiner's office. Oklahoma City Chief Medical Examiner Dr. Fred Jordan and his colleague Dr. Larry Balding welcomed me and showed me into their autopsy suite, where the mysterious leg was waiting.

"It's up to you now, Emily," Barry told me. "I'll check back with you in about an hour and see how you're doing."

I took a deep breath and thought for a moment of the 168 lives that had been lost in the bombing, and of Timothy McVeigh and Terry Nichols, who were now in custody and charged with that crime. Then I put all thoughts of crime out of my mind and began examining the leg. Until I had finished this task, I was solely and purely a scientist.

•   •   •

The Oklahoma City case had begun on the morning of April 19, 1995, when hundreds of people were busy inside the Murrah Federal Building. Some of them were federal agents, but most were civilians, working for federal agencies, mopping the floors, or maybe even filling out applications for those jobs. Visitors in the building were applying for Social Security benefits or filling out passport applications or dropping their kids off for a day of supervised play at the day-care center housed in the building's front corner.

Then, at 9:02 a.m., a massive truck bomb exploded just outside, destroying the building. Emergency teams launched a massive rescue and recovery effort and managed to evacuate hundreds of injured and frightened victims, but after the dust settled, 168 people were still unaccounted for, including 19 children. Fifteen of those children had been at the day-care center. The other four had been inside with their parents.

An investigation of the crime began immediately, even as the medical examiner started an all-out effort to find and identify the bodies and body parts that remained within the building. Meanwhile, the FBI called in the forensic anthropologists at the Smithsonian Institution and AFIP. This was, after all, a terrorist act and a mass homicide, so the FBI's concerns went way beyond simply identifying the victims. They wanted to recover and document every piece of evidence so that they could use it to prosecute whoever was responsible for this terrible crime.

The medical examiner's office also had the services of Dr. Clyde Snow, a world-famous forensic anthropologist who had served for many years as their consultant. When the widely respected Dr. Snow wasn't in South America investigating the deaths of "the disappeared"— victims of the death squads in Argentina's political wars in the 1970s— he was handling cases for the medical examiner, and he began working nonstop to help identify the victims. With the invaluable assistance of the entire medical examiner's staff and local rescue workers, investigators had managed to recover and identify all but three of the victims by the end of May.

When I heard about their efforts, I had a sudden image of how painful the death analyses on those victims must have been. Many of the people investigating these deaths lived in and around Oklahoma City—as did the victims. Very likely, the people dealing with the remains were looking at the torn and broken bodies of people they knew—colleagues, neighbors, friends. I had never had to perform an autopsy on someone I had even met, let alone become close to, and I could only imagine how painful such an experience would be.

By the end of May, recovery workers had pulled so much rubble out from the base of the bombed-out building that engineers felt it wasn't safe to continue digging. They believed that the bodies of three victims still remained in the building—but the only way to get them out was to implode the building, to avoid the danger of it collapsing on the rescue workers. Then workers would dig their way through the rubble to recover the remaining bodies. Of course, the imploding building might further damage the remains. But that was a chance they would have to take.

Although they couldn't reach the bodies, investigators already had a pretty good idea of where they were. So on May 29, they applied some brightly colored spray paint to the area they could reach and backed out to allow the engineering experts to bring down the rest of the building. Hopefully, the spray paint would help lead them to the right portion of the rubble once the building went down.

And indeed it did. After the implosion, rescue workers quickly found the three remaining bodies and pulled them from the rubble. At the bottom of this massive pile of rubble they also found a portion of a decomposed leg. But no one could match this leg to any of the bodies that had already been recovered.

•   •   •

Meanwhile, the search for the perpetrators had continued. Within two days of the bombing, an observant state trooper pulled over a yellow Mercury because it didn't have a license plate. The driver, Timothy

McVeigh, was arrested about eighty miles north of Oklahoma City and put in the local jail for a number of reasons unrelated to the bombing: because he didn't have a license plate, or proof of insurance, or a license for the concealed pistol the trooper spied hidden under his arm. Just moments before McVeigh was scheduled to be released on bail, investigators sharing information via state computer links connected him to the Oklahoma City bombing, so his jail time was extended until the FBI could explore this connection. Soon a federal grand jury had indicted McVeigh for the bombing of the Oklahoma City Federal Building.

People who knew McVeigh described him as a white supremacist and advocate of the right-wing militia movement. Investigators soon concluded that McVeigh was responsible for the bombing—but he hadn't done it by himself. Police eventually arrested and charged Terry Nichols, another alleged white supremacist and militia supporter.

McVeigh was headed for trial, where his team of lawyers was likely to suggest that yet another person had been involved in the bombing—a man who soon became known as John Doe #2. Before McVeigh was arrested, the police had found an axle from the rented Ryder truck that had held the bomb. They managed to link the truck to a Ryder rental agency in Kansas, where they interviewed the rental clerks involved. Clerks told police that they thought they'd seen two men together. John Doe #1 turned out to be McVeigh. But who was the mysterious John Doe #2? It probably wasn't Nichols. He reportedly was hundreds of miles away at the time. So McVeigh's lawyer tried to suggest that this third man—who has not been found to this day—was the real mastermind behind the bombing, with McVeigh and Nichols merely his pawns.

Then lead defense attorney Steven Jones found out about the mysterious "extra leg." In his book about the trial, *Others Unknown,* he claims to have made this discovery by accident, sometime during the summer, when an Oklahoma state trooper leaked the information to him. Jones, in turn, leaked the story to the *Dallas Morning News* and to

Time magazine. *Time* publicized the fact that an "extra" unidentified leg existed and, suddenly, this body part became the focus of a nation-wide controversy.

Jones claimed that the leg could be helpful to his case, as it might have belonged to the "real" architect of the Oklahoma City bombing. According to him, federal prosecutors had deliberately—and improperly—withheld from him information about this leg, which he argued belonged to a White man wearing military combat gear.

In fact, the forensic experts had initially thought that the leg was from a White man, but they weren't absolutely certain. They weren't being evasive—they simply couldn't tell for sure. Since the limb had been discovered, it had been analyzed first by experts in the Oklahoma City medical examiner's office and then by FBI specialists from Washington, D.C. At both levels, forensic scientists found a certain amount of ambiguity in the evidence that caused them to revise their findings.

A few things were certain. Experts determined that the leg had been traumatically amputated about six inches above the knee—presumably by the explosion itself. They also found evidence that the limb had been very close to the epicenter of the initial explosion. Blue plastic shards, which looked as if they might have come from the blue plastic drums that held the explosives, had been driven deep into the bone by the force of the blast. The foot was dressed in two pairs of dark socks and a black combat-style boot, with a military-style blousing strap at the top of the boot—the kind of device used to secure the cuff of a soldier's trousers.

The clothing certainly seemed more likely to be worn by a man than by a woman—but some women do wear combat uniforms. The bone data seemed ambiguous as well: the leg might have come from either a robust woman or an average-sized man. Anthropologists commonly depend on the statistical probability that men's bones are larger than women's, but because of the variations inherent in humankind, these probabilities are little more than good statistical guesses. There are no hard-and-fast rules that can positively divide the sexes based on bone size alone.

Sometimes you can use other indicators, but they're not terribly reliable. Death investigators will duly note whether leg hairs have been shaved—but not all women shave their legs, while some men do. Polished toenails are a more reliable indicator of sex, although many women don't paint their nails—and again, some men do. In this case, the initial evidence did not add up to a single, definitive picture of this individual's sex.

Nor could investigators be certain about race. The leg had been damaged from the blast and was partially decayed. Since it had lain in the rubble for several weeks, its skin had already decomposed somewhat and begun to discolor. The skin was generally light-colored—but did that indicate that the body was Caucasian or only that the epidermis had sloughed off? Some areas of the skin were slightly darker than others—but was that from natural pigmentation or darkening due to decay?

Although investigators could see the leg's skin color for themselves, they understood that such visual cues are a highly unreliable indicator of racial identity. Color often changes during the decay process, and in our multicolored United States, people of all different hues identify as "White" or "Black," with some White people's skin visibly darker than that of people who call themselves African American.

Since the evidence was ambiguous, the Oklahoma City experts released inconclusive results, finding that the leg had probably belonged to a Caucasian, with a 75 percent chance of its being male, and a 25 percent chance of its being female. But they also sent tissue and hair samples to FBI specialists in Washington, D.C.

The FBI experts began to revise the initial results, though they, too, were reluctant to issue a definitive report, given the ambiguity of the evidence. The FBI's tests concluded that this individual was probably not male but female, not White but Black.

Their findings were based on a number of factors, including the dark hairs found on the leg. But they knew very well that it's hard to determine a racial identification from leg hairs alone—scalp hairs tend to be a more reliable indicator. Of course, if the leg hair had been naturally blond, they could probably have concluded that the person was Caucasian. But people of all races have black or dark-brown leg hair.

Had the leg not been amputated, they might have been able to look at the anterior curvature in the shaft of the femur, which, as I had learned in grad school, is a fairly reliable indicator that can be used to separate Whites and Blacks. In this case, though, the femur stopped just above the knee. Then Dr. Ubelaker and Dr. Snow remembered the paper I had written on racial elements in the bone structure of the knee—and that's where I came in.

•   •   •

Meanwhile, the defense was making as much as possible of the leg's discovery. Thinking they might be able to blame the entire incident on this enigmatic leg, they began very early in the investigation to refer to it as the leg of the "real bomber." They went back to the initial reports about John Doe #2—who had been reported as a husky dark-haired man wearing a baseball cap. This mystery man, the lawyers argued, was the culprit who deserved the death penalty, not their client.

Jones and his defense team built up an elaborate defense based on this mystery leg. First, they pointed out, the leg had been found at the epicenter of the blast—the most likely place for the "real bomber" to be. Second, the initial forensic exam had indicated that the leg had probably belonged to a White male—the most likely profile for such a bomber. Since the bombing seemed to be the work of white supremacists and militia supporters, it seemed highly unlikely that either a Black person or a woman would have been the "real bomber" in such a crime—if only because it was so unlikely that McVeigh would ever have taken orders from anyone other than a "superior officer," who in the ranks of the right-wing militia would most likely be a White man.

Thus, when the FBI issued their second opinion, suggesting that the remains were more likely those of a Black female, the defense called this a transparent attempt by the federal government to win its case against McVeigh. The FBI's laboratory analyses were under particular scrutiny because, ever since the O. J. Simpson case, whistle-blower Dr. Frederick Whitehurst had been accusing the Bureau of falsifying laboratory results in favor of prosecutors.

Besides, the defense pointed out, the leg couldn't be linked to any of the victims who had been recovered and identified. If there was in fact an "unknown" victim, he or she must have been someone who didn't belong in the Federal Building—further suggesting that the leg belonged to the "real bomber."

So a great deal of the case came down to the mysterious John Doe #2, the husky dark-haired White male in a baseball cap whom several witnesses had claimed to see with McVeigh in the days before the bombing. The defense was doing everything it could to prove that this leg belonged to John Doe #2, while the prosecution was working hard to prove that it didn't. The defense seemed to be ready to accuse the prosecution of falsifying results so that it could cover up the identity of the "real bomber" and convict McVeigh in his place.

That's why determining the race and sex of this leg became such an issue. A high-level group of people, including Clyde Snow and experts from the medical examiner's office, the FBI, and the Smithsonian, held a daylong meeting to determine their next course of action. At the end of that day, they called me at my office in Frankfort, Kentucky.

Dr. Doug Ubelaker, the FBI's top forensic anthropology consultant at the Smithsonian, explained the problem. He'd just read my article in the *Journal of Forensic Sciences* announcing my discovery of the racial variation in the intercondylar notch of the femur. After he'd discussed my research with the others, they all agreed to invite me out to Oklahoma City to apply that theory to their mystery leg. The FBI would pay all my expenses—but they needed me as soon as possible.

Of course, I was flattered and said I'd do what I could to help. After checking with my employer, I called back the next day and agreed to fly out. After just a few hours in the air, I got to the medical examiner's office and was first introduced to Dr. Larry Balding, the Oklahoma City forensic pathologist who had done most of the analysis of the parts found in the building, and the one with whom I would be working.

I had enormous respect for him, Chief Medical Examiner Dr. Jordan, and of course Dr. Snow—all of these people were heroes in my eyes, and I thought it might be a bit unnerving walking into a strange morgue and working with them on such a high-profile case.

But the sounds and smells of the morgue were reassuringly familiar. I'd been on staff in Kentucky for more than a year, and by now an autopsy suite was home ground. I spent a grueling but satisfying day examining every inch of the leg, analyzing tissues, measuring x-rays, and taking detailed handwritten notes.

As the day wore on, Dr. Balding, Barry, and some of the other FBI agents began hovering over my shoulder, eager to hear some preliminary conclusions. I was reluctant to do my standard "thinking out loud" until I was pretty sure of what I was seeing, though, because this case was complicated and controversial enough already. The last thing I wanted was for one of these high-level people to take down a premature conclusion and begin to run with it, only for me to have to tell them at the end of the day that I had changed my mind.

But by the end of the afternoon, I was ready to go on the record. I called the other investigators together and shared my opinion that this leg had belonged to a woman—a woman who was undoubtedly Black. At this early stage in my investigation, I told them, much of my conclusion was not based on peer-reviewed research. Rather, it grew out of my experience of observing thousands of knee reconstructions and repairs on athletes from all racial groups, and from dissecting and analyzing literally hundreds of amputated legs at the Hughston Clinic. However, just as I had that late night in Dr. Bass's lab at the University of Tennessee, I just *knew*.

Of course, in my written report I'd follow Bass's teachings and limit my conclusions to facts and figures that would stand up in court. Even so, I had enough solid scientific information to corroborate the FBI's determination that this individual was female, with a significant amount of Negroid ancestry. We agreed that I'd return to the morgue the next morning to continue documenting my findings. By the next afternoon, I'd be flying back to Kentucky.

Barry offered to drive me to my motel, and as soon as we were on the road, we returned to an engrossing discussion of this case that fascinated both of us. I was looking straight at him, absorbed in my explanation of why I could only include the scientifically sound material in my written report, leaving out the impressions I got from feeling and seeing subtle contours in the bones, ligaments, and menisci.

Suddenly, out of the corner of my eye, I saw a flash of blue—then my head and shoulders whipped left and then right—and then things simply went dark. Either I blacked out from the force of the whiplash, or else I'd closed my eyes in reflex. The next thing I saw was open air on our right as we teetered on the brink of an overpass while the huge tractor-trailer rig on our left slammed against us a second time, ripping into the steel at Barry's shoulder.

By now Barry's car was up on its right side, skidding along on two wheels, and I was looking straight down into what seemed like an abyss. I just knew we were going to die.

The screech of metal on metal seemed to go on forever as we were shaken back and forth, crunched between the truck on one side and the guardrail. Finally, Barry managed to maneuver the car back to an upright position, locking it under the chassis of the semi's trailer. The truck continued to drag us along until we were off the bridge, where we broke free and stopped. The truck kept rolling for several yards until it, too, managed to stop.

The driver of the truck had gotten out, approaching us with an aggressive swagger. Then Barry put his blue light on the dash and pulled out his FBI badge. The trucker's posture changed immediately, and he headed back for his truck. As he walked away, I noticed with a shiver that he was a husky man with dark hair, wearing a baseball cap. The local police took over from there, and I don't know what happened after that.

Luckily, neither Barry nor I was seriously hurt, but my right arm was bruised and swollen. By morning my neck was stiff and sore, and my head ached so much that I had to cut short my plans to complete my report before I left town. Though I hadn't liked to give in to my suspicions, some of the folks at the morgue started teasing us, hinting that Barry and I had been deliberately targeted by the "others unknown"—the mysterious heroes of those who enthusiastically believed that the bombing had been the work of a huge and powerful team of conspirators determined to bring down the federal government, one piece at a time. Since Barry was one of the key investigators and I was there to cast doubt on the identity of the leg, we were logical targets.

I didn't put too much stock in the teasing and neither did Barry. Still, I was glad to get on the plane for Kentucky that afternoon. I'd had enough for one day.

Later, when Jones published his book, he criticized the Oklahoma City medical examiner and the FBI for having the temerity to send a young, inexperienced, recent graduate to help sort out the case. I found his description ironic—I think Jones and I are about the same age and, of course, at that point I'd had nearly twenty years experience analyzing amputated human legs and skeletons. He was right about one thing, though: I *was* a recent graduate.

Jones also wrote that he submitted my report to Dr. Bernard Knight at the Royal Infirmary in Wales. According to Jones, Knight was skeptical about my report, concluding that the leg had to be from the "real bomber."

Knight was wrong, however, and by February 1996 Dr. Jordan and the FBI were able to prove it. Once the forensic experts were certain that the leg belonged to a Black female, they were able to confirm it was the left leg of a young African American woman named Lakesha Levy.

Lakesha was a twenty-one-year-old Airman First Class at nearby Tinker Airforce Base who had been killed in the blast while applying for a Social Security card, leaving her husband a widower and her five-year-old son without a mother. Her body had been identified during the first few weeks of the investigation and she was now buried in a New Orleans cemetery—with someone else's left leg.

The authorities were able to get the other leg exhumed and return it to the Oklahoma City medical examiner's office, where experts were trying to identify it. The initial mistake was understandable. Mass fatality incidents usually involve significant destruction of soft tissues and commingling of bodies and body parts, so unless someone makes a concerted effort to separate all human remains at the site, this type of separation must be done with precision at the morgue.

In this case, an unattached or "unassociated" left leg from someone else had mistakenly been linked to Lakesha at the crime scene, an error that had somehow slipped by at autopsy. The human body is simply not designed to withstand the physical forces that come from massive explosions or collapsing buildings; such powerful energies tear bodies apart and mangle the remains, making it extremely difficult to determine what belongs to whom.

That's what had happened to Lakesha and the owner of this second leg. Although this other mystery leg was still unidentified by the time McVeigh went to trial, examiners now almost universally agreed that the leg mistakenly buried with Lakesha had once belonged to a White female. The defense team tried to suggest perhaps this second leg had belonged to the "real bomber," but by now this theory had lost a lot of credibility. If simple human error had caused the first mix-up, it seemed likely to be responsible for the second, as well.

Nevertheless, after McVeigh's conviction, Drs. Jordan and Balding asked me to return to Oklahoma City to examine this second leg. My analysis simply corroborated their opinion that the victim was a White female.

My second trip to Oklahoma was an opportunity to work with and stay with Dr. Snow and his wife in the nearby town of Norman. Dr. Snow shared with me how devastating it had been for him and his colleagues to deal with such a tragedy there on their own turf. The community was so small, he told me, that almost everyone had a personal connection to the bombing. It had been painful enough dealing with the families of the "disappeared" in Argentina, but coping with this kind of event in his own backyard was overwhelmingly sad.

I left Oklahoma City with a powerful sense of sorrow, as I thought of the murders I dealt with in Kentucky and the mass fatalities I'd seen in Waco and Oklahoma City. It all seemed part of a terrible cycle of violence, especially since most investigators believe that the Oklahoma bombing was at least partially an act of revenge against the federal agents who had laid siege to the Branch Davidians at Waco. My work had given me a painfully close look at the kind of people who tried to force people and governments to accept their values by violence—and an even closer look at the shattered lives they leave in their wake.

8

World Trade Center

From a proud tower in the town,
Death looks gigantically down.

— EDGAR ALLAN POE

WHEN THE bus let me off in front of the morgue in New York City, I was struck by a powerful sense of déjà vu. I had first come here on September 23, 2001, in response to the attack on the World Trade Center, so that I could help identify the thousands upon thousands of human remains that the disaster had caused. I had worked a relentless schedule of twelve-hour shifts for thirty straight days until, finally, my tour of duty ended and I went home. Now it was November 18, and I was back for my second tour. I felt as though I had never left.

I showed my pass to the police officer, and he waved me past the barricade, toward the huge tent city that had sprung up on Manhattan's

Lower East Side, beside the city's central morgue and the Office of the
Chief Medical Examiner (OCME). Here, morgue workers examined
the bodies and body parts that had been extracted from the rubble,
identifying some, analyzing the rest, and storing the unidentified
remains so that, hopefully, one day they could be returned to their
grieving families. The people working here were law enforcement
specialists, evidence technicians, forensic medical scientists, and full-
time OCME personnel, as well as volunteers from all over the United
States—but they were also New York beat cops, detectives, SWAT
team members, and police clerks, pressed into service to handle a volume of death and destruction that the city had never known and that
involved many of their own fallen comrades.

I headed down the street, ignoring the refrigerator trucks in which
the newly arrived body bags were stored and the tents where people
handed out food and toiletries and sweatshirts. I thought only of how
I could reach the morgue in time to relieve the workers who had been
working nonstop for the past twelve hours. Then I noticed the ambulance with its flashing lights and the two dozen police officers who had
just come out of the morgue to greet it. The police stood silently as the
ambulance doors opened and a flag-draped body bag emerged. On
command, every officer snapped to attention, saluting as paramedics
lifted the bag onto a stainless steel gurney.

I went to stand among them, feeling the comfort of their presence,
my right hand over my heart in a civilian salute. NYPD Sergeant Mark
Giffen stepped over to the gurney, the silence broken only by the endless city traffic that rushed up First Avenue behind us. He folded the
flag, handed it to Captain Marilyn Skaekel, and added his salute to the
rest. "At ease," she said finally. Six of the police officers, each wearing
hospital scrubs, sprang into action, pulling back the tent flaps that covered the morgue's entrance, wheeling the gurney inside, and opening
the bag so that Amy Zelson Mundorff, the forensic anthropologist who
ran the day shift, could begin to examine its contents.

I hurried on past the morgue to the small yellow-and-white supply
tent—crammed to overflowing with scrubs, plastic gowns, and latex

gloves—and suited up like the rest. In less than five minutes, I was back in the morgue, where autopsy tables and portable carts full of medical instruments lined the walls. However, the initial examination was already complete, and a morgue worker was hand-delivering the contents of the body bag to the x-ray technician.

Mark Grogan, a young Irish cop with flaming red hair, looked up from the clipboard, on which he'd been taking notes as the forensic pathologist dictated his findings. Mark rose to his feet immediately, throwing his arms around my shoulders in a long tight hug. He never said a word, but I knew he knew. So did the others. We had worked together for every night of that first long month and we had become true comrades in arms. Soon after I'd left that first tour of duty, Mark had called me at home, and through uncontrollable tears I'd told him that my father had died of cancer just hours before his call. Dr. Reuben Craig had been my hero, my fishing partner, my mentor, my rock, my dad. And now he was gone.

Mark released me from his hug and I took a long grateful look at the other members of my triage team as they prepared to start the night shift. It's hard enough facing a death that comes after a long, lingering illness—but at least you have time to say good-bye. When death happens suddenly, violently, on a grand scale, there's an extra sense of outrage, an anger at the senseless loss that unites not only the survivors, but also those of us who deal with the victims. It was this bond that had kept me going on my first assignment to New York, and it was this bond that I was seeking once again.

Amy and I completed the routine business of a daily shift change, and I took my place in front of the next body bag, my hands already feeling through the torn flesh. I realized that something very important had changed. Before, despite my sympathy for those who'd lost their loved ones, I'd been able to keep some measure of the scientific detachment that had served me so well at the countless death investigations I had handled over the past ten years. Now, the loss of my father had opened something new in my heart, a grief that echoed the public mourning around me, an agony that flowed straight into my hands.

As the night-shift workers gathered around me, ready to begin another night of processing the dead, I thought perhaps that they, too, could sense the difference.

·   ·   ·

Like everyone else in America that morning, I woke on September 11 with no idea of how profoundly that day would affect my life. The night before, I'd gotten a call about some skeletal remains discovered in an isolated wooded area out by Bowling Green, Kentucky—remains that the coroner thought might be those of a fifteen-year-old girl who had been missing for two weeks. Halfway to the scene, I idly flipped on the radio, and what I heard sounded more like a disaster movie than real life. As the hysterical announcer explained that an airplane had slammed into Tower 1 of the World Trade Center, I cranked up the volume, unable to believe my ears. Then I heard about Tower 2.

I wanted to turn the van around and go home, where I could watch this horrifying event on television and wait for the call from the Disaster Mortuary Operational Response Team (DMORT), a national volunteer operation I had joined about three years before. Whenever there's a disaster that goes beyond the resources of a local area, DMORT mobilizes mortuary workers and death investigators from around the country to help pitch in. They'd called me in to help with other mass-fatality incidents and I couldn't go, so I desperately wanted to be in the first wave of response to this shocking event—to do something, anything, that might counteract the helpless rage that was suddenly welling up inside me.

But all I could do was keep driving. Like every other rescue worker in America, I was anxious to spring into action and help wherever I could, but I knew that the isolated Kentucky crime scene was in a valley beyond the reach of cell phones. DMORT would surely be trying to reach me—and when they couldn't, I knew they'd go on to the next name on their list.

When I finally got to the crime scene, I felt as though I'd entered the twilight zone. There was none of the banter, the easy camaraderie that death scene investigators rely upon to help us cope with our morbid tasks. Instead, we were all in shock—partly because of the horror that always overtakes a death scene when a child is involved, partly because of the larger tragedy that none of us knew how to process. I felt as though we were all going in slow motion, and I was amazed, the first time I checked my watch, to see that, in fact, we were proceeding at normal speed.

I'd called in forensic specialists from halfway across the state to meet me at the crime scene, and as they arrived they would each try to describe the devastation they had watched on television that morning. But even those who had seen the footage with their own eyes had a hard time believing what had actually happened. Each person who arrived brought further news. The nation's airports had been shut down. Terrorists had attacked the Pentagon. A plane had gone down in Pennsylvania. The president had been whisked into hiding.

Here in the woods, an eerie quiet surrounded us. Because all aircraft had been grounded, there was none of the usual noise from planes flying in and out of the nearby airport. Even the police radios—usually crackling nonstop at a crime scene—were silent, since everyone had been ordered to keep the airwaves free for emergency communications. One of the deputies would periodically drive to where he could get a phone signal, call his dispatcher, and bring back additional bits of news.

I tried to imagine the falling buildings, the thousands of lives snuffed out. I had never even seen the Twin Towers in person, but my mind returned obsessively to the scene again and again.

When I finally got back to my lab in Frankfort, I found my voice mailbox full of messages and my e-mail crammed with urgent requests from DMORT. But when I called the regional commander, it was just as I'd feared. They'd wanted to send me, but they'd had to move on. They would surely be calling me later, the commander told me—but, for now, they had all the help they needed.

Back at home, in front of the television, I felt a wave of dread. Now that I could actually see the Twin Towers come down, I understood from experience something that many others didn't realize right away—there would be almost no survivors. And the remains of the victims would be mangled almost beyond recognition, mixed in with steel and concrete and rubble. As at Waco and Oklahoma City, but on a much larger scale, the recovery effort would involve pulling shredded body parts out of a mass of debris and then somehow trying to identify the remains as part of a leg, a shoulder muscle, a kidney. It was just the kind of work I'd been doing for the past ten years, and I knew that very few other people would be willing or able to do it. Because of my odd, checkered career—all the time I'd spent dissecting remains at the Hughston Clinic; the months of memorizing bone fragments at the University of Tennessee at Knoxville; and the many fires, explosions, plane crashes, and homicidal dismemberment cases I'd worked in Kentucky—I had somehow put together precisely the combination of skills that would be useful in a situation like this.

I settled down to watch yet another replay of that morning's horrifying disaster. Whether or not I was part of the first response team didn't matter anymore. Sooner or later, I knew, I'd be going.

•   •   •

The first few days following the attacks are a blur. As I tried to keep up with events in New York, we identified the teenaged homicide victim from Bowling Green and managed to determine the cause of her death. I did my best to finish up the rest of my active cases so that when DMORT called for reinforcements I'd be ready. As I'd suspected, all three disaster sites were soon flooded with volunteers; but, with the airports shut down, even DMORT had great difficulty getting enough workers to the New York and Pennsylvania sites (the damage to the Pentagon came under the jurisdiction of the military and other federal agencies). Nevertheless, the logistics were still an enormous challenge. DMORT command had even sent some people to military bases, with instructions to travel by military transport. Those volunteers waited endless hours in cold hangars, spending the night on cots—only to learn that military resources were needed elsewhere and they'd have to drive for two days to get to their destinations.

DMORT was fearful, too, of putting a huge percentage of the nation's forensic experts in one place. What if our entire team of forensic experts, mortuary specialists, and medical death investigators were all sent to New York and then someone blew up their hotel or staged another attack in the recovery area? And what would happen if there were then new attacks in other cities?

Neither DMORT nor any other U.S. agency had ever dealt with a disaster of this magnitude. Before DMORT came on the scene, only two agencies dealt with mass disasters—incidents in which the number of dead is beyond the resources of a local community. The Federal Emergency Management Agency (FEMA) supervised rescue and recovery operations during earthquakes, floods, hurricanes, and tornados, while the National Transportation Safety Board (NTSB) responded to train wrecks, airplane crashes, and other transportation-related incidents.

These agencies did admirable work, but there were some gaps in the services they provided to the families of the deceased. DMORT evolved as a way of supporting those who had lost loved ones in mass-fatality incidents, making sure they got the information they needed and providing them with social services. Gradually, the agency began to add other forensic specialists to their team of funeral directors and mortuary experts, including medical personnel; forensic anthropologists, pathologists, and odontologists; fingerprint specialists; dental and x-ray technicians; and DNA analysts—resources drawn from all over the country to supplement the personnel available in any one location. Likewise, DMORT recruited such skilled workers as heavy-equipment operators, security specialists, photographers, and investigators, as well as administrative support staff, computer specialists, and the like.

Eventually, a protocol developed for integrating DMORT into disaster relief. The first step, obviously, is always to deal with the living casualties. When the Federal Building went down in Oklahoma City, rescue workers were pulling survivors out of the wreckage for days. Emergency disaster relief focused on bringing additional doctors, nurses, and medical personnel—anyone who could deal with the needs of the wounded.

Once the living are taken care of, attention can be paid to the dead. The second wave of disaster personnel is the forensic specialists who can perform autopsies on corpses, match their recovered teeth to dental records, compare fingerprints, and analyze fragmented body parts and bone shards. That's usually where I come in—sometimes days or even weeks after the initial disaster.

.   .   .

On the evening of September 22, I finally got the call. DMORT wanted me to fly out the next morning and report to their New York City headquarters in the LaGuardia Marriott, a large hotel near New York's LaGuardia Airport. The authorities had first planned to set up morgue operations in an airplane hangar there, so DMORT chose a nearby location to house their staff. When that plan changed, we all moved to a midtown hotel, about a week later; but meanwhile, here I was, walking into a lobby that seemed so deserted I wondered if I had come to the wrong place.

It seemed that the hotel had moved all of its regular guests to other quarters so that DMORT could commandeer almost the entire facility. The hotel staff was basically serving only rescue workers, and they approached me with a subdued readiness to help that I think they saw as their contribution to the recovery effort.

I appreciated their concern as they directed me to my room and then showed me how to follow the arrows that had been taped inside elevator doors and at every landing, directing me to "DMORT-MST." MST stood for "Management Support Team," the administrative wing of DMORT. Whenever there's a disaster, MST is there, arranging for the living quarters, food, telephone lines, computers, faxes, photocopiers, and all the other necessities that nobody notices—unless they're not there. Now, MST staff helped me fill out all of the necessary paperwork and signed me up as a temporary employee of the U.S. Department of Health and Human Services (DHHS), part of their National Disaster Medical System. (In the summer of 2003, this division became part of the Department of Homeland Security.) As a member of their team, I'd be paid an hourly salary and receive a per diem allotment to cover food and incidentals. The hotel room was free, courtesy of my new employer.

Being in DMORT is a bit like being in the National Guard, although in our case response to an incident is strictly voluntary. We keep our regular jobs, but when the country needs us to serve somewhere, we work things out with our bosses and go. My superiors at home had agreed to bring in anthropologists from neighboring states to cover any routine cases that might arise, as long as I promised to come back if I were truly needed.

Over my three tours of duty in New York, I tried my best to keep up with my Kentucky commitments. When I was on the night shift, signing in at six p.m. and checking out at seven a.m., I made sure never to sleep past four p.m. so I could use that final hour of the normal workday to return calls to my home state. Then, sometime between two a.m. and four a.m., when there was usually a lull in activity at the morgue, I'd answer my office e-mail—courtesy of the library at nearby NYU Hospital, which had offered us their computer services. So even while I was serving DMORT in New York, I was still keeping up with my job in Kentucky: examining digital pictures of bones e-mailed to me by coroners (thankfully, all were nonhuman, or I might have had to go back); corresponding with detectives about active cases; and working with attorneys to arrange my scheduled testimony for upcoming trials. Because I was still working for the Commonwealth, I still had to fill out my time sheets, answer the many questions routinely called in by police and families, and otherwise provide the kind of ongoing presence required by my office.

All of us in DMORT had gone through a rigorous application process and, once we'd been accepted, we had to attend mandatory

annual training sessions. Although I'd had plenty of experience working in emergency situations, this wasn't true for all the funeral directors, dentists, and other volunteers who'd come to DMORT from
private practice, and it was important for us all to learn how to work
together as one cohesive unit. For people used to being their own
bosses, it was important to learn how to take orders, work under strict
federal guidelines, follow protocol, and make the shift from dealing
with individual patients to working on a virtual assembly line of people, living or dead. Those of us who dealt primarily in law enforcement
had our own lessons to learn: how to develop working relationships
with other types of professionals; finding ways of building trust and
camaraderie and mutual respect. The last thing you want in an emergency situation is any kind of turf war.

Of course, people being what they are, there *were* turf wars, among
us workers at the bottom and all the way up to the agency heads at the
top. But by the time I came on the scene, ten days into the crisis, a lot
of the interagency battles had already been sorted out.

．　　　．　　　．

At five forty-five the next morning, I walked into the hotel dining
room that MST had reserved for our twice-daily meetings and immediately felt like part of the team. This kind of briefing was familiar from
my days at Waco, though there were almost three times as many people at these meetings, and there was still more pressure to move quickly
and cooperatively. It helped to be dressed like everyone else; all of us
DMORT personnel were wearing standard-issue battle-dress uniforms: khaki shirts with button-down flap pockets, multi-pocketed
pants, high-topped black combat boots—uniforms that made us
instantly recognizable and helped us function as a unit amid the firefighters and police officers.

The businesslike briefing left little time for greetings and socializing.
At six a.m. sharp, DMORT Region 4 commander Dale Downy started
in with a quick report on the recovery efforts at the three terrorist tar-

get sites, relaying the latest words of encouragement from President Bush and DHHS Secretary Tommy Thompson. Then he gave us our assignments. I was going to the morgue to help with triage.

As I boarded the chartered bus that would take me down to the morgue, I couldn't quite picture what was in store. Despite my experience in multiple-fatality incidents, I'd never dealt with anything remotely like this—none of us had. In other cases, the scope of the disaster had seemed finite. We'd had some kind of list of who the victims were, records that enabled us to match remains to names. Here, the chaos seemed endless and so did the tragedy.

I was riding with a group of mortuary workers who had been in New York from early on. These old-timers leaned their heads against the windows and either stared into the dark or tried to nap, while a few of us newcomers talked quietly, trying to diffuse some of the nervous anticipation that became more intense the closer we got to Manhattan, our nerves keyed up by the flashing blue lights and whining siren of the police escort that led our way.

We arrived at the morgue just as the sun was coming up. The night-shift workers were anxious to board these same buses for the ride home and they'd gathered in the street behind the police barricade—groggy, dirty, with sightless, glazed-over eyes. They tried to greet us with encouraging smiles and handshakes, but I could tell they were exhausted.

I allowed my colleagues to sweep me along as we crossed the police barricade at First Avenue and funneled through the checkpoint set up by the New York State Police at the end of the block. The morgue was down 30th Street, half a block away.

Security was tight here, and each of us had to show our DMORT identification badge to two uniformed officers. Then I followed the other members of the team down this street toward the East River, into the tent city that had been set up within hours of the disaster to analyze and identify the remains of what was then assumed to be more than five thousand victims.

The OCME had commandeered the entire area, and I looked

around quickly, trying to get the lay of the land. In the middle of the block was the garage-type entrance to New York City's permanent morgue, on the ground floor of a six-story brick building that handled the "routine" violent and accidental deaths in this huge city. Within hours of the disaster, Chief Medical Examiner Dr. Charles Hirsch had realized that his regular autopsy suite would hardly be enough, and he initiated his agency's mass-fatality plan—turning his building's delivery garage into the disaster morgue and tacking on a three-sided tent, which extended our work space right down to the street. Heavy reinforced plastic flaps let us seal off the disaster morgue entrance tent from rain, wind, or cold, though the flaps were almost always left open to allow air to circulate and the typical morgue odors to dissipate. Despite the disaster, New York City's regular forensic business had to continue, so the standard autopsy suite and the modified emergency morgue operated side by side as parallel worlds—one for routine violence, the other for disaster.

I came to think of the left side of the street as the medical section of Tent City. First came two refrigerated trailers, the kind normally pulled along the highway as the back part of a semi or tractor-trailer rig. These trailers, known as "reefers," were attached to large diesel-powered refrigeration units that periodically roared to life as they tried to keep the trailer's contents cool. Here, workers stored the body bags as they were brought in from the disaster site so that we could process the remains in a steady stream, rather than allowing them to stack up and deteriorate in the heat of the day.

To the right was the "support side" of the street—another group of white tents whose yellow- and blue-striped roofs lent an incongruous circus air to the area. I noticed a chapel, complete with altar, flowers, and rows of benches—a private yet communal place where the rescue workers could share a moment of much-needed quiet. Then there was a tent stacked with mysterious-looking cardboard boxes, which I later found out contained such personal items as toothbrushes, soap, shaving supplies, even packages of underwear and socks—anything that displaced workers might need when they had to work here for days at a stretch, without time for a long commute back to the suburbs.

The next tent was filled with police officers. When I saw some of them standing around drinking coffee and smoking cigarettes, taking a brief break from the urgent pace of work, I felt the urge to smile. I was finally starting to feel at home.

Then there was the morgue, whose open tent flaps allowed a clear view all the way inside. I saw six stainless steel autopsy trays, each long enough to hold a human body, supported by a pair of sawhorses. Behind each tray was a stainless steel cart filled with latex gloves, marking pens, plastic bags of all sizes, scissors, knives, and a bone saw.

A team of medical specialists surrounded each tray, moving in the highly synchronized choreography that you see in an operating room, an ER—or a morgue. The noise was overwhelming as the workers shouted to one another over bone saws that whined like dentists' drills. Clerks wearing hospital scrubs stood by, passing labeled folders to the pathologists each time a new body bag was loaded onto their table. And over it all hung the heavy smell of death, along with diesel fuel from the nearby reefers.

I wanted to stop for a closer look, but my colleagues were making their way to the tent labeled DMORT. Inside, their twenty-by-twenty-foot nylon tent was crammed so full of people and supplies that there was barely room to move. The side walls were stacked with boxes of disposable surgical gloves and gowns, while along the back were paper towels, notebooks, and office supplies. I noticed some military-issue canvas cots where exhausted morgue workers might catch a catnap during breaks, and in the center of the tent were a half-dozen folding chairs surrounding a makeshift table—a large wooden spool normally used to hold a coil of steel cable. It remained me of something you'd have at a fishing camp.

This table held the sign-in sheet that each of us had to initial each day before we scattered to our various assignments. The DMORT supervisor on duty, Cliff Oldfield, knew that this was my first day, so he told me to stand by. In just a few minutes, he promised, he'd tell me everything I needed to know.

When Cliff brought me over to the morgue, Amy Zelson Mundorff, the forensic anthropologist who worked full-time for the city's chief medical examiner, was ready to greet me. I saw immediately how personal this tragedy was for her and her colleagues—although she was smiling brightly, large purple and green bruises ringed her eyes, and her forehead sprouted a lump large enough to cast a shadow. Cliff had told me that she, along with Dr. Hirsch and several other OCME staff members, had rushed to the Twin Towers shortly after the first plane hit. They were in the process of trying to establish a site for a temporary morgue when Tower 2 had come crashing down. The blast blew her headfirst into the marble pillar of a nearby building, while Dr. Hirsch escaped death by inches. One staff member suffered a massive concussion and fractured ribs, and another's leg was shattered, leaving bone and muscle exposed to the air.

However, Amy, just barely five feet tall and sporting a head full of curly black hair, was still very much alive and eager to get on with the business of victim identification. After she gave me a whirlwind tour of the medical examiner's office, we wound up at ground level in the morgue tent, where she took her place at the first autopsy table, the one designated for triage. As she worked, she quickly explained the overall recovery and identification protocol.

The protocol we were using was based on the emergency plans that the OCME had developed well in advance of September 11, with modifications that Dr. Hirsch had added when the scope of the disaster became clear. This protocol fascinated me: It was both different from and similar to the setup at the other incidents I had worked.

Most mass-fatality morgues are set up in sort of an assembly-line format. Rescue personnel bring in bodies or body parts to be photographed, x-rayed, and preliminarily identified by careful scrutiny of superficial characteristics such as hair color, skin color, clothing, and perhaps jewelry.

If the body is relatively intact, the forensic pathologist will conduct an exam that is not too different from normal autopsy protocol. He or she will photograph, weigh, measure, and describe the body in painstaking detail, including observations on its overall condition and any old scars or other evidence of surgery that the preliminary exam might have missed. The pathologist will also document the acute injuries that most likely caused the person's death—documentation that would eventually include photographs and a detailed written or dictated description.

In some cases, as in the Oklahoma City bombing, living perpetrators are involved who may eventually stand trial for murder. The medicolegal details of autopsies might well have ramifications for their criminal prosecution.

But the attack on the Twin Towers was a completely different situation. There was no reason to conduct traditional medicolegal autopsies: Millions of people had witnessed the events as they happened. We all knew that these were deaths by homicide and that none of the hijackers could have escaped alive. It would be virtually impossible to identify the specific causes of death for each victim. All that mattered was identifying the victims themselves—but that task was difficult enough.

Here, the first step in the identification process was triage, a French word that means "to separate." The term is used primarily in battlefield or medical situations, where patients or victims are separated into categories based on how urgent it is to treat them. This triage process began with a forensic anthropologist who had to identify and separate every single bit of human tissue that came through the morgue door. If a bag came in filled with a twenty-pound mass of muscle, skin, and bone, we had to be able to tell either by feel or by sight if the tissues were connected. If a bone led to a tendon, and then to a muscle, and the other end of the same muscle was connected to yet another bone, then the entire specimen could stay together and be processed as a single set of remains, because the "connections" established the fact that these were the remains of one person. But if we determined that there was no physical connection between one part and another, then we'd separate the remains and give them two different case numbers. Hope-fully, DNA analysis could later link the two, but for now we kept them separate.

Triage could also reunite body parts. If we found two ends or sides of a fractured bone in this mass of tissue, the broken surfaces of which we could match or "reapproximate," then we could say with all confi-dence that these two pieces were from the same victim. Our ultimate goal was to match all of the remains with a name, but much of that would come later, through DNA analysis.

Sometimes, an entire body arrived. More often, we had to sort through mangled remains—shards of bone, shredded flesh, the frag-ments and pieces that remained after the conflagration—identifying them as best we could.

Once an anthropologist had completed that first step, morgue work-ers carried the remains over to the pathologists working at the other end of the morgue. These men and women assigned each body or body part a case number, examined the tissue, and collected samples for DNA analysis. Morgue staff would then label the samples. They had already started an individual case file on each body or body part, doc-umenting everything we did with it along with everything we could find out about it.

An escort then took custody of the tissue, making certain that the body or remains arrived wherever the pathologist thought they should go next. Perhaps the fingerprint expert could provide further help in identifying a finger or a hand, or the dental identification unit might analyze a tooth that had emerged intact. Maybe an x-ray could deter-mine whether a bone or bone fragment revealed previous evidence of breaking or surgery. Any of these steps might be crucial in ultimately identifying these precious remains.

When the specialists had finished their analysis, an escort would hand-deliver the remains to Memorial Park, where everything was stored pending DNA analysis. Hopefully, that analysis would ultimately enable these bodies and body parts to be returned to their grieving families. Meanwhile, a huge team of investigators upstairs at the medical examiner's office was busily trying to match the reports from the pathologists with the missing persons reports, hoping to get results to the families even before the DNA results came back.

When I met Dr. Hirsch, we soon discovered that he was a close friend and colleague of our own Dr. Hunsaker, with whom I'd worked on my very first Kentucky case. The connection made us feel like friends and, although Dr. Hirsch, too, was working nonstop, he took the time to escort me down to Memorial Park, an enormous storage facility created in only a few days to store the dozens of victims and tens of thousands of body parts created by the disaster.

Dr. Hirsch and his staff had commandeered a vacant lot by the East River, which they had paved in asphalt. They brought in sixteen refrigerated trucks, similar to the ones at the morgue entrance, and had them parked side by side in two parallel rows of eight. Then workers erected an enormous white tent that soared forty feet into the air. The effect inside was that of a large cathedral, an awe-inspiring sight.

When Dr. Hirsch opened a door to one of the refrigerated storage trucks, the chilled air took my breath away and temporarily fogged my glasses. The temperature had to be kept close to freezing to preserve these fragile samples as long as possible. As my vision cleared, I could make out shelves lining the walls from floor to ceiling, stacked with plastic bags and boxes full of body parts. Intended as a temporary facility, Memorial Park is still in existence at the time I write this, as DNA analysis of the remains continues.

•   •   •

Back at the morgue, I watched the triage team for several hours, trying to take in all the details and learn the protocol. I saw how well choreographed the triage was, how every staff member knew exactly what to do and when to do it, in a seamless rhythm that reminded me of the first time I'd watched an operation.

The next day began in the same way: first the briefing, then the bus ride at daybreak. By the time I got to the morgue, I already felt like an old-timer—so much so that I found myself speaking up during triage. "Oh, that's got to be the flexor tendons of the forearm," I heard myself say.

Amy looked around, startled. I had been standing behind her so quietly, I think she'd almost forgotten I was there.

"Where do you see that?" she asked, half taken aback, half amused at my temerity.

The whole team was staring at me over their protective masks. I swallowed hard and replied as calmly as I could:

"Well, that thin band of parallel fibers looks like the flexor retinaculum, and I can see a fragment of the wrist's pisiform bone still embedded in that tendon over on the side. That tendon is running at a right angle to the retinaculum. So unless I miss my guess, you should be able to reach in and straighten out those other tendons and the attached muscles, and then tease out bits of the median and ulnar nerves running right along with them."

Amy looked over at me. The corners of her eyes crinkled over the top of her mask, and I could only imagine that she was smiling.

"Thanks, Emily." Then she dropped the bombshell: "I think you'll be ready to handle the night shift on your own if you keep this up."

What? I had just arrived on the scene a few hours ago, and they were going to put me in charge of triage for the night shift?

Amy, I knew, was running the day shift, working twelve hours a day, seven days a week. Dr. Dawnie Steadman, from Binghamton in upstate New York, was managing the night shift now, but her tour of duty was supposed to end in one day. If I was up to speed, I'd be taking Dr. Steadman's place. I still couldn't quite believe I was being put in charge so soon. But my training as both bone specialist and anatomist had served me in good stead to start the triage process by identifying each mix of bones and soft tissue that came through our door. If OCME and DMORT thought I was ready, well, then, I'd be ready.

· · ·

"So, Emily, how are you making out?" Amy asked during our next break.

"I think I've got the basic sense of things." However, it was still hard for me to grasp how some bodies had emerged intact from the blast while others were reduced to amorphous balls of rubbery gray tissue, how incinerated bones could be found next to a piece of skin with an intact tattoo.

"It will all make more sense to you if you go down to Ground Zero," said NYPD Captain Kenneth Mekeel, who was standing there with us. I hadn't yet begun to learn people's names, but there was no question that this man was in charge. Mekeel supervised the law enforcement officers working the day shift, and coordinated the flow of human remains between Ground Zero and the OCME. He also coordinated communication with the site at Staten Island, which I would learn about later that afternoon. The gold bars on the captain's shoulders and the row of medals on his chest broadcast his rank, but it was his quick, confident way of speaking that told me he was not only used to giving orders, but also used to having them obeyed. And he was easy to spot in the crowd, which was a great help. Whenever anyone came by asking where the captain was, they were just told to look for the crisp white shirt on the man with the ramrod spine.

"I'll see if I can find someone to give you a ride down to Ground Zero and a Cook's tour," he offered now.

Like just about everyone else in the country, I had an almost primal need to see Ground Zero. For days I had been watching television coverage of the event, and every reporter on the air had said that unless you actually saw it for yourself you just couldn't comprehend the extent of the catastrophe. They were right.

Mekeel arranged for an FBI agent to come pick me up in his car, and we drove down there with another FBI agent who, like me, had just arrived in New York the day before. On our way downtown, everything seemed surprisingly normal. The streets were full of people going about their business, shopping or on their way to work. As we got closer to the site, though, the whole atmosphere began to resemble a ghost town: the streets blocked off, the police cars not even bothering to use a siren as they raced up and down the deserted avenues.

Even FBI agents weren't allowed to drive their cars onto the disaster site, so we parked several blocks away and walked up to one of the checkpoints guarded by military police. As at the morgue, we each had to show two forms of picture identification and to sign in. "Make sure you exit through this same checkpoint and sign out on the same logbook," the guard warned us. This was both a matter of security—restricting unauthorized personnel—and of safety, making sure that everyone who went in came out again safely.

Mekeel had let me borrow his hard hat and safety goggles, which I donned just like everyone else on the grounds. Even so, we were limited to the outer perimeter of the site—which was just fine with me. It was hectic and dangerous enough where we were.

The forces that had wrenched and burned the steel were almost beyond comprehension. The air was filled with smoke that carried the unmistakable odor of burning human flesh, and everywhere I looked I could see piles of pulverized concrete and other debris. On the smoldering piles of rubble closer to the center, I saw a hellish whirlwind of smoke and ash swirling over mountains of concrete rubble, glass, and structural steel beams. The gigantic size of these buildings started to register in my imagination—even their collapsed remnants dwarfed the huge grappling cranes that had been brought in to help remove the debris, and the workers scrambling back and forth across this eerie landscape looked like tiny insects.

On the edge of sixteen acres of devastation, we, too, were dwarfed by the massive trucks of all shapes and sizes that rumbled past. Some were bringing in supplies and equipment to help with the recovery effort. Others were military troop transport vehicles filled with rescue workers. Tanker trucks came in loaded with fuel for the cranes and bulldozers—and, of course, fire trucks and other emergency vehicles carried men and women who were trying desperately to contain the fires still raging in the belly of this monster.

"Monster" was not too strong a word, I thought, watching the pile of debris belch fire. It almost seemed to be moving of its own accord as the wind whipped any flexible object back and forth while loose pieces of the buildings' skeletons lost their grip and crashed down, sounding like thunder when they landed. Whenever any person or object touched the ground, huge clouds of gray dust billowed up and seemed to stay suspended indefinitely, first rising, then blowing back and forth in response to the bizarre combination of air currents created by the fires, the wind, and the trucks whizzing by in all directions.

It was impossible to hear anything over the machinery, so the three of us communicated by hand signals. As my FBI "tour guide" signaled me to follow him, he also pointed downward, indicating that I should watch where I stepped. I looked down and saw that the ground was covered with a matrix several inches deep—coarse sand, glass, bits of electrical wires, and large sections of twisted steel. To my horror, I also saw bits of bone.

I shouldn't have been surprised. Bone fragments as well as body parts had flooded the morgue all morning long and, now that I had a better idea of the magnitude of the destruction, I knew in my heart that these fragments might be all that was left of many of the lives lost on that terrible morning. An overwhelming sadness entered my heart, and I had to fight hard to hold back tears. I was literally yanked back to attention when someone grabbed my arm and pulled me out of the way of a Humvee coming toward us in reverse at breakneck speed. The driver, in camouflage, a helmet, and goggles, barely glanced in our direction as he maneuvered his vehicle up onto the deserted sidewalk and continued on his way.

As we got closer to the site, I was struck by the intense, determined activity of the recovery workers. The devastation seemed huge—yet you could feel that the people here wouldn't rest until they'd cleaned it up. Huge cranes and other heavy construction equipment dug into the massive piles of material, while firefighters and Port Authority officers scanned the mass of twisted metal and concrete with a sharp eye out for any evidence of human remains. Whenever anyone spotted a body or body part, he or she would wave to equipment operators to halt immediately. Then one lone man or woman would move in, crawling over the mountain of debris to gently extract the remains and put them in a bag. If someone found a whole body or a large recognizable section of a body, he or she would store it in a conventional body bag—but very few of those were needed. (By the time I left my third tour of duty in January, the final count of whole bodies recovered from the site was slightly more than two hundred.) The remains were more likely to fit into two-by-two-foot red plastic bags or even small freezer-size plastic zipper-lock bags.

We continued to walk around the entire site, over to where Coast Guard boats were patrolling the river, past a makeshift memorial to the victims—one of hundreds that had sprung up all over the city—then past a parking garage still filled with cars that had been parked there on that fateful morning. By now, they were all coated in a thick layer of the sand-like debris that also covered the streets and sidewalks, as if some volcano had erupted and showered everything with ash. We stopped for a moment in a small church that seemed to have escaped damage even though it was frighteningly near the destruction's epicenter.

Firefighters and other rescue personnel were scattered across the rows of pews, some sitting quietly with their heads bowed, some on their knees in prayer, and others walking up and down the outer aisles gazing at the pictures and handmade posters taped to the walls— desperate messages from the victims' families and friends, pleading for information and hoping against hope that the person in the picture had somehow made it out alive. I couldn't look. I knew then and there that the only way I could do this job was to insulate myself from the names and faces there on the wall. In that instant, I surrounded myself with the invisible defensive cocoon that I had spun from experience and kept hidden in my soul for such times. I knew that now, more than ever, my private wall was the only thing that would make it possible for me to deal with this overwhelming human tragedy.

It had been years since I had prayed inside a church, but I stepped up to the altar, lightly placed my fingertips on the cross, and shut my eyes. When I finally looked up, I turned on my heels and headed for the door with a new sense of purpose. As I headed back to the morgue, I now understood that I *had* to do this job. Not for myself, not for DMORT—but for the victims and the people who loved them.

•   •   •

On the way back, my FBI guide explained to me the third leg of the recovery effort, one that I'd never actually see for myself but which was an integral part of the work I would do here. When human remains were spotted in a particular place at Ground Zero, he explained to me, they were recovered and sent uptown to the OCME disaster morgue. Then, workers excavated the rubble and debris from that same location and sent it over to the Fresh Kills landfill at Staten Island on barges. Trucks on Staten Island off-loaded this material and workers spread it out on the ground so they could examine it once again for any traces of human tissue. Indeed, some body parts were so small or so camouflaged by their coating of pulverized concrete that they slipped by the spotters at Ground Zero and were only separated from the rubble at the Staten Island facility.

Eventually, forensic experts from around the country worked around the clock for more than eight months on Staten Island, separating bone and flesh from more than sixty-one million tons of shattered metal and concrete. By the last few months of the effort, they had created a huge assembly-line operation with conveyor belts and commercial sifters. They'd also built a semi-permanent tent city that offered the workers some shelter from the weather, housed the cafeteria and a dining area, and served as space for office work and evidence processing.

As I returned to the morgue, I realized that my vision of the disaster had shifted. Before, I had been looking for an explanation of why the results of the towers' collapse were so horribly uneven—how a relatively intact body could lie side by side with a tiny bone fragment. But once I saw the magnitude of the destruction, I realized that there was no point in seeking such answers for the mechanisms of injury. We just had to accept things as they were and deal with the results.

And soon it would be my turn to deal with those results on my own. Today was Wednesday. On Thursday I'd be taking over the night shift triage station in the morgue. I had only tomorrow to get ready.

·   ·   ·

On Thursday morning, I didn't get up and go to the morgue with the day-shift workers. Instead, I tried to adjust my sleep/wake schedule by taking a few naps and keeping the room dark and quiet. I'd be expected to show up at the six p.m. briefing that evening and be ready to go as if it were the start of a normal work day—and then I'd be in the belly of the morgue until seven the next morning.

As I lay in my hotel room bed at two o'clock that afternoon, the thought of having to go to sleep when my built-in diurnal clock was telling me to wake up was almost more than I could bear. I punched the pillow, turned over, and tried to will myself into a state of relaxation. Tonight, I'd face the test.

·   ·   ·

When I walked into the morgue that night, the first thing I did was run through a mental checklist of the guys on my team, the men and women I'd met over the past two days who would be helping me with triage. To my Kentucky eyes, they were an almost archetypal group of New Yorkers, colorful and brash. Al Muller, a detective with the NYPD, was our company jokester, always ready to crack a smile and find something funny in even the most awful situation. Mickey was a Port Authority cop who reminded me of a quick-witted and quick-tempered jockey I once met at Churchill Downs. Carmen was part of the NYPD's missing persons unit; an exuberant Latina, she switched back and forth between Spanish and English without even thinking about it. A police officer, Mia, was a headstrong diva with long black dreadlocks and a swagger to her walk. Kam worked on the NYPD Emergency Response Team—a man of action whose skin was the color of oiled mahogany. Mark Caruso was the first openly gay police officer I'd ever met. He complained endlessly—but he was always the first to come up with a pep talk when we needed it, laughing at everything and everybody. Just to make me feel a little more at home, there were Mark Grogan and Don Thacke, the New York versions of the Kentucky and Tennessee cops I'd come to know and love.

And then there was John Trotter: my buddy, my comrade in arms, my right-hand man.

John was a Port Authority detective who shaved his head bald as a cue ball but cultivated a thick white beard. A big, broad-shouldered John Wayne kind of guy, he'd gone down to the World Trade Center right after the first plane hit, trying to get his people out. When Tower 2 started to come down, he ran for his life with a bunch of his men. He zigged and they zagged—so he survived and they died, even though they were all within inches of one another. John was down there, too, when the fighter planes roared over the area, and he didn't know if the planes belonged to friend or foe. All he knew is that he and the civilians he was shepherding out of the area might once again be in danger of death.

After all he'd been through, John felt that he couldn't go back down to the site to help with rescue and recovery. But he'd been on the job for thirty years, and his bosses knew they had to find something for him. So he'd ended up assigned to the morgue, and I never had a better helper in my life. He seemed to get totally absorbed in the work, as though knowing that he was doing something vitally important for the victims' families and friends—not to mention his own fallen comrades—gave him a way to cope with his own loss. He became a darned good anthropologist, too, recognizing bones almost as quickly as I did, and sometimes helping me figure out which bone some of the fragments belonged to.

John and I were about the only middle-aged ones among a big

group of twenty- and thirty-year-olds, and I think we each appreciated not being the only "old-timer." We offered each other moral support when the hours and body parts at our table seemed endless, and we often hung out together during breaks.

Although John and I shared a special bond, every single person on my team was steady, faithful, and smart. I adored them and I would have trusted them with my life. And I was honored—and relieved— by how quickly we all seemed to put our faith in each other.

My team was already experienced in the carefully choreographed procedure that kept the identification process running like the assembly line it was. Mickey brought me my first body bag and unzipped it, revealing that it contained a smaller plastic bag. Al reached in and removed the bag, then read the tag telling us where it had been found. Steve, another member of my team, removed the tag and reached under the table for a new bag, while Al cut the first bag open. Then John reached over and removed whatever was inside, handing it to me. I did my best to tell what it was and to see if there was anything in or on it that might help with identification. More often than not, my "identification" was limited to saying that the body part was a tip of an elbow, or a section of lung, or maybe a fragment of mandible, but sometimes we would open a body bag that contained almost an entire torso or even a complete body.

In most mass-fatality incidents, such as high-impact plane crashes, the only materials you can use for a positive ID are teeth, bones, unique tattoos, fingerprints, or DNA. People often think we can use associated evidence—an article of clothing or an ID card—but that's only good for a "presumptive identification": The body or body part that accompanies it must still be identified by scientific means.

In a few rare cases, you can use objects to make a positive ID. If a unique ring is found on someone's finger, the hand can be ID'd—but that's no help with the victim's other body parts if they aren't connected. Or if the human remains contain a surgical device that bears a serial number, you might use that for a positive ID. But most other personal effects don't help you identify a body part because they can so easily become commingled: These effects, along with parts of the victims themselves, are often inextricably mixed with one another. Watches and other jewelry can actually be torn from one victim and recovered from directly on top of or under another victim.

So, back in the morgue, if we found a unique and identifiable watch securely circling the wrist of a severed arm, we were able to make a tentative ID of the entire upper extremity, but the pathologist still had to take a DNA sample in hope of eventually linking that arm to the rest of that victim's remains.

It's always difficult to identify human remains after a mass disaster. A small plane crash or a minor industrial mishap—even a house fire or a space heater's explosion—can shred a human body, mingling remains with rubble. I'd worked a number of such scenes in Kentucky, and my primary objective had always been to find a body part that might ultimately be used to make a positive ID. Maybe I'd pick up a single fingertip torn from the rest of the hand—the basis for a fingerprint that might later be matched to a coffee cup left at home on the breakfast table. Or I might find a small piece of skin with a unique tattoo, or a gold-capped tooth torn from its socket that could eventually be matched with a dental record.

That process of sorting and identifying human remains is hard enough in an "ordinary" disaster, when you've got a dozen or a hundred victims to deal with. But nearly three thousand? All of whom had died either in the plane crashes, the fires, or the collapse of the buildings—from one of the several forces that had reduced a gigantic steel-frame structure to rubble?

Yet, I reflected, watching the swift and precise movements of my team and the pathologists' team on the other side of the morgue, human bones and teeth are incredibly durable. Their mineral content is made up primarily of calcium hydroxyapatite crystals, so they can often withstand the fires of commercial crematory retorts that can reach as high as 2,300 degrees Fahrenheit. And bones shattered by bullets and motor vehicle collisions can often be screwed or pinned back together well enough to allow them—and their owners—to survive happily for decades.

Now these sturdy bones were being brought into the morgue by the thousands. And it was up to us to identify them and send them on for further analysis. So after I had named whatever I could recognize, Mark or Mickey would write my description on the new bag, into which John or I would gently place the tissues in question. One of the other morgue workers—Audrey, Terry, or Vinnie—would carry the bag over to one of the pathologists, who had their own group at the other end of the morgue, close enough for us to work together but far enough to avoid DNA cross-contamination from the various body parts. The pathologists were technically in charge of the whole operation, but they worked as members of the team, assigning case numbers, dictating detailed descriptions of the remains, instructing Diana to take x-rays, Joe or Raoul to take fingerprints, or a dentist to analyze the teeth. They took the DNA samples themselves. Barbara, the Port Authority sergeant, was there, too, helping things to go smoothly.

Meanwhile, at my end of the morgue, I felt my way through the mangled remains, trying to come up with some bone or a recognizable bit of soft tissue to which I could give a name. I had the unmistakable sense of everything coming together again—the dissections I'd done in Georgia; the work in Texas, Tennessee, and Kentucky; the years of memorizing bone fragments in Dr. Bass's osteology class. Here I was using all of it—and the stakes had never been higher.

On and on I worked, my hands seeming to move of their own accord, my mind automatically naming and noticing and cataloguing. Every once in a while we'd get a body that was relatively intact, perhaps one that had been sheltered by fortuitous physics as the structures imploded. Somehow, the combination of kinetic forces had formed a few pockets that denied access to the pulverized concrete and debris. While the victims found here died just as suddenly as the others—their lives snuffed out quickly from the heat, lack of oxygen, and explosive pressures of the implosion—their bodies were not torn asunder and they could be returned in relatively recognizable shape to their grieving families, having been identified by standard means—dental records, fingerprints, and/or unique tattoos.

Mainly, though, we were working with fragmented and unassociated bones or body parts. But although we were moving at a relentless pace, the mood in the morgue wasn't tense—instead it was somber, almost reverent. Every single one of us was aware that the remains we handled were all that was left of somebody's loved one, that a fingertip or bone shard might be all that a family would have to mourn over and cherish after such a sudden loss of life.

Indeed, the remains we handled might well belong to someone that my triage team had known personally—one of John's Port Authority buddies, or a colleague of Mark's from the force. Usually, in a morgue, you have complete detatchment—the morgue workers are rarely acquainted with the people who have died, and that impersonality is as important to us as it is to a surgeon, who can make a healing incision on a stranger that he or she could never make on a parent, child, spouse, or friend. Yet even though in Kentucky we *did* occasionally work on people we knew, the far greater likelihood that my New York team could at any moment encounter a colleague or buddy created a sorrow that hung in the air as palpably as the smell of death. Every single one of us handled every single body part as though it had belonged to our own father or mother, our own child, brother, sister, or spouse. Each of us treated these shattered bits with respect—and maybe even with love.

Despite the very personal grief that these police officers felt, they worked with an unfailing commitment and caring that never failed to move me. They were there by my side the whole time, opening bags, transcribing the words I was using to describe the tissues: "right distal femur," "left foot," "portion of scapula." At first I had to spell some of the technical terms I was using, but in spite of my southern drawl, they soon caught on to what I was saying, and since we were seeing so many of the same bones I no longer had to spell out m-a-n-u-b-r-i-u-m when I identified a fragment that had come from the top of someone's breastbone.

These guys not only helped me with the logistical problems of identifying and re-bagging the remains, they helped me stay focused. It was easy to get emotionally involved with the work—a piece of monogrammed jewelry around a neck or a name badge still pinned to a victim's shirt constantly drove home the fact that these weren't just shattered bodies, they were also shattered lives. We all did our jobs efficiently and with care, but sometimes the stress got to be too much and we had to stop, step outside the tent, and get some fresh air just to clear our heads.

When I started that first night, I was especially serious. After all, I was the new girl in town and I was well aware of how personally everyone took this work. And my trip to Ground Zero that afternoon had fired me with my own sense of reverence for the remains I handled. Hour after hour we focused on our jobs, with barely a superfluous word or unnecessary comment. I'm sure my team members wondered how they could stand to work with me for the next two weeks if this unbroken seriousness was all that was in store.

Then, right before midnight, something broke through the shell of the ultraprofessional demeanor I had assumed to cover my nervousness. Al opened up a small red biohazard bag containing a flat piece of mangled tissue. Gently, I teased it apart so that I could get a good look at it, dictating notes about the muscle mass and the little bit of white fat around the edge. But when I caught sight of the splinter of bone, I looked up from my delicate task, gazing at John, Mickey, and Al in turn.

And then I started to laugh.

Everyone was shocked. Being super-serious might not be acceptable, but laughing at a dead person's body part? What kind of monster was I?

I reached down, grabbed the piece of bone, and waved it in front of them. "It's a pork chop!"

There was a moment of silence. Then we all started to chuckle— quietly, so the pathologists on the other side of the room wouldn't think we had all gone crazy.

"How in the heck did *that* get in here?" I asked.

Mickey knew the answer. "There were restaurants in and around the Twin Towers. In fact, during the first day or two after the attack, we found part of a side of beef inside one of the body bags."

I shook my head. "At least no one expects us to catalogue *that*."

That wasn't the last time I encountered nonhuman tissue. Throughout my time in the morgue I managed to catch a good number of chicken bones, beef ribs, and even a few legs of lamb before they were given case numbers.

Other laughs were few and far between inside this morgue. The solemn care with which we tried to handle even the smallest fragment of tissue often threw a mantle of despair over us all, and when we got a respite between shipments of body parts, we would gather in the street or inside one of the adjacent tents or trailers and tell stories of life away from death. The cops from New York delighted in telling me about life in the Big Apple, and I, in turn, would reveal some of my adventures in the hills of Kentucky. They teased me about my accent and I made fun of theirs. I taught them how to say *"y'all"* with just the right inflection—and I couldn't wait to get back to Kentucky and greet folks with *"How you DOin'?"* just as my teammates taught me.

·　　·　　·

When I first started working at the morgue, I was continually amazed by the tent city that had sprung up around it, and by the generosity and creativity of the New Yorkers who were trying to show their support in any way they could. Just around the corner from us, the Salvation Army and numerous charitable organizations made sure we had a continuous supply of soft drinks, water, candy, and crackers, as well as hot meals three times a day. The Salvation Army canteen was staffed continually and offered not only good, nourishing food, but smiles and a touch of home. Their tables often had fresh flowers in little bud vases and notes from schoolchildren and other well-wishers taped to the walls. Someone had obviously put a lot of thought into the decorating scheme, because these notes were positioned throughout the makeshift dining hall, so that wherever you looked, you could see someone's message of hope or thanks.

When I first got to New York, the weather was balmy, but when it got cold outside, the Salvation Army brought kerosene heaters into the mess tent. A common sight inside the dining tent was a group of morgue workers clustered around one of these devices, holding out hands that were chilled and raw from repetitive washings and hours inside thin latex gloves. The bustle and camaraderie of tired workers in surgical scrubs working long hours, combined with the makeshift surroundings, made the whole thing look like a scene out of the TV show *M★A★S★H*.

•   •   •

One of the hardest parts of my New York tours was how disoriented my life became. Working on the night shift meant that I practically never saw the daylight. I'd leave for work at six p.m., when it was already dark, and return home at seven a.m., when the sun had not yet quite come up. And when you work all night long for more than a month, you begin to lose all sense of time. The hours blend into one another and so do the days, because every day is exactly like the one before and the one you know will come after. It's hard on a practical level—how do you manage to do your laundry, or get a haircut, or call your niece to say "Happy Birthday"? But it's hard on a psychological level, too—a sustained course of sensory deprivation and lack of sunlight that I found almost as wearing as the pervasive grief.

One day, though, my routine was broken—though not necessarily in a way I would have chosen. Late one afternoon near the middle of October, DMORT regional commander Todd Ellis made an urgent call to my room, telling me to go immediately to the command post that filled the top floor of the Sheraton New York Hotel, where we were now staying. Lieutenant William Keegan, the night shift recovery supervisor at Ground Zero, needed my help recovering some incinerated bones on top of what they now called "the pile"—the mountain of debris that had once been the Twin Towers.

Until recently, several fires had smoldered in and around the pile, and firefighters had only recently managed to put them out. As a result, searchers were just now starting to gain access to this area, a mass of rubble and concrete that rose up steeply, supported only by the enormous steel beams that had somehow survived the blast. As soon as workers had seen the burned bone fragments, they halted that particular excavation effort until I could get there and help with the bones' removal.

Two uniformed NYPD officers rushed me to the site in a nerve-wracking trip: speeding through the streets of New York in a police car with flashing lights and a siren that pierced the air, skirting other vehicles and pedestrians with only inches to spare. Finally, we reached our destination, the battle-scarred face of Engine 10 fire station, where Lieutenant Keegan was waiting for me. Quickly, he led me to an area where dozens of police officers were sifting through buckets of fragmented concrete, searching desperately for the bones of their fallen brothers.

"We found a weapon and a charred NYPD badge up there by that grappling crane, so we know at least one police officer was up there," Keegan explained. "But we're not sure how to get the rest of the bones out without any more damage." He pointed almost straight up, past a bulldozer and a huge crane that now seemed to be poised in mid-swing. Their diesel engines were rumbling at idle as the operators sat quietly, watching the sifters down below.

"We'd like you to come up there with us," Keegan continued. I wished I could say no—but how could I refuse? With my heart in my throat, I inched my way up the face of the pile, gripping the slabs of broken concrete and picking my way carefully across pieces of steel that spanned cavernous spaces below. I looked down once into a seemingly bottomless abyss, where glowing embers from somewhere below sent up tendrils of smoke that stung my eyes. I tried not to look down again—but looking up was almost as frightening. The steel framework that had formed the towers' façade rose to incredible heights in front of me, and I could swear that it seemed to move. Then, I realized that it was actually the ground that was moving, in what felt like a sustained minor earthquake, a subtle shifting and an almost constant vibration of the materials under my feet.

"That movement is from all the heavy equipment working on other sections of the site," Keegan explained. "This whole mass of debris is sort of suspended like jackstraws, so when one piece shifts, sometimes the whole thing moves."

"Oh, boy," I said to myself. "I thought all those days spent in sink-holes, coal mines, and limestone ravines back home had made you tough, Emily. But this is almost too much for the old girl." I bluffed myself past my fear and kept going.

I'd taken to heart Keegan's sense of emergency, so the moment I reached the top of the pile, I began suggesting to the cops and fire-fighters what I thought we should do. Almost immediately, I could see, they began to get their backs up, rolling their eyes and muttering to each other. But I'd been in this situation before, though, and I had some idea how to handle it.

"Now, gentlemen," I said, with just a hint of smile and my best Southern drawl. "I know you are all experienced rescuers. After all, you are New York's Finest and Bravest, and I'm nothing but a blonde from Kentucky. But I think we can level the playing field here a little if y'all call *me* 'Doc' and I call *y'all* 'Sugar.' "

After a shocked pause, they burst out laughing, and that was all it took. For the next hour, we sifted bones out of the ash, working together as colleagues. They taught me how to recognize artifacts buried in the odd assortment of debris we were digging through, and I taught them how to recognize fragments of calcined bone.

.   .   .

A standard DMORT tour of duty is two weeks long. After my first two weeks were up, DMORT asked me to stay for a second tour and I readily agreed. Then, a few days before my second tour of duty

ended—when I would have served thirty nights without a break—
DMORT asked me to stay on for a third tour.

"I just can't do it," I told my commander. "I haven't seen daylight in
four weeks. I'm brain-dead, I'm exhausted, and I have a mountain of
work waiting for me back in Kentucky. Please, cut me my orders and
send me home." What I thought but didn't say was that I was also emotionally wrung out. As the head of night shift triage and one of the
older workers on-site, I was the person on whom the others had
leaned. They counted on me to keep it together when someone burst
into uncontrollable tears or wandered outside in a daze, overcome by
the realization that the remains on the table belonged to a person he or
she had known. I was more than willing to provide any support I
could—but now I simply had nothing left to give.

My commander agreed to send me back to Kentucky with the
understanding that I'd be called later and asked to return to New York.
I didn't say anything to anyone, but I guess the word spread. My last
night of that first month, when we hit a little lull, Carmen said, "Oh,
Doc, we've got one more bag here that we missed somehow." Wearily,
I unzipped it—and there were two ceramic angels and a card that
everyone had signed. As I hugged and kissed every single one of my
amazing colleagues, I wondered if I'd ever find the strength to return.

·　·　·

When I got off the plane in Kentucky the next afternoon, I felt dazed
and bewildered. This was home, and it was so familiar. But I'd been
away for a month, and I'd seen and done things that would change me
forever. It felt strange and disorienting to be without my "combat buddies," the men and women with whom I'd worked side by side on a
job that, I now realized, I'd never really be able to explain to anybody
else. We'd shared something that only made sense to those of us who'd
been through it, and now I had no one to share it with. I was looking
forward to seeing my friends and talking with my family—but I also
felt terribly alone.

My first stop on the way home was Daisy Hill Kennel, where my beloved springer spaniel had spent the past month. I hated to leave Savannah in a kennel, even for a short time. But my neighbors Suzanne and Bill Cassity had introduced me to the people at this long-term animal facility right before I'd left for New York, and I felt confident that my pet would be well cared for there. To my amazement, when I went to pick her up, I found notes and letters from strangers who had left not only words of encouragement for me and my colleagues, but also enough money to pay my kennel bill.

I had managed to stay in control for the past four weeks, but now, driving home with Savannah by my side, I felt my emotional walls start to crumble. As soon as I got home, I collapsed, sobbing on my bed as Savannah tried desperately to lick the tears off my cheeks. Life and love were proving to be stronger than death, and I surrendered to a wave of overwhelming sadness as I held Savannah tightly to my chest and allowed her soft fur to soak up my tears.

I fell asleep after this cathartic cry but was wrested awake a few hours later by a ringing telephone. It was my mother, telling me that Dad was close to death. If I wanted to see him again, she told me, I should come to Indiana right away. I'd known my dad had cancer, of course, but when I left for New York City, we'd all thought he was holding his own. Soon afterward, he began a rapid decline, which he and my mother decided to keep secret from me as long as I was in New York. Only months later did Mom tell me that, by sheer will alone, Dad had held on until I got home.

So, the next day, Savannah was back at Daisy Hill and I was back on the road. I spent ten days in Indiana—long enough to say goodbye to my dad, who slipped into a coma the day after I got there. Two weeks after I'd gotten back from Indiana, I returned to New York for my next tour of duty—and I was glad to be there. Maybe staying focused on the city's enormous loss would help keep my mind off my own sorrow.

·　　·　　·

When I took the taxi from LaGuardia Airport into midtown the afternoon of November 18, I was struck by how much had changed. When I'd arrived in September, the whole city had seemed subdued. Although I had little opportunity to interact with any civilians other than the workers in our two hotels, I had the sense that in the first few weeks after the disaster, New Yorkers were treating one another with special gentleness and care. The few times I managed to stretch my legs in a walk around the block, the famous New York City crowds seemed to graciously make way for me, as though no one wanted to be guilty of a careless shove or a brusque "Out of my way." I barely even heard a honking horn.

On this return trip, the whole mood of the city seemed different. Traffic seemed faster, more impatient, and definitely louder. Things seemed to be getting back to normal in this bustling, overcrowded city, which I supposed might be considered a good thing.

It wasn't so good for us DMORT workers, though. Our work had always been hard, but now it seemed to be discouraging—and lonely as well. Sometimes it seemed that we were the only ones who knew what was going on behind closed doors while the rest of the world was understandably busy with getting back to normal, even preparing for the holidays.

But the friends and families of the victims were there with us, if only in spirit. They knew that we were working around the clock, and they still hoped that at any moment we would find and identify someone they loved. It was hard on those days when we couldn't and gratifying on those days when we could.

Like my first tour of duty, my second started as a fourteen-day assignment and ended up as four straight weeks—including Thanksgiving. Since none of us got holidays off, the Salvation Army had prepared Thanksgiving dinner for us in their tent, so during a break between shipments from Ground Zero, John Trotter and I made our way through the food line and found seats in the back, near the heater. The golden September days were long over, and the end of that November day had turned cold, rainy, and dreary. I was grateful for the heat and for the cheery attitudes of the Salvation Army volunteers who served us. They seemed almost apologetic that they didn't have better food to offer us, but I saw nothing wrong with the turkey, mashed potatoes, sweet potatoes, and green beans that they heaped on our plates. Slices of cold white bread were a poor substitute for hot rolls, but several homemade pies had apparently been donated to the workers at the Ground Zero site, and someone had thought to scrounge a few desserts for us folks behind the front lines.

The food was fine, but this was a far cry from the Thanksgiving dinners that John and I were used to, happy occasions that we usually spent with family and friends. Now we were alone and far from home—but at least we had each other.

"I love having you here for company, Emily," John was saying. "But I wish I was at home."

I was almost more upset seeing John's pain than feeling my own. John had seemed to grow much older since I'd first met him in September. He had lost some of that sturdy enthusiasm that I so valued in him, and now he talked often of retirement.

At nine o'clock on this rainy Thanksgiving night, John and I were the only people who were eating dinner, so we basically had the place to ourselves. Shortly after we'd carried our trays back by the heater, the volunteers up front dimmed the lights and huddled into their own little conversation group to pass the time until their next "customer" arrived. A minute later, one of them came back and placed a candle in the middle of our tiny Formica-covered table, then backed away without a word. I couldn't help but think about that classic scene from Walt Disney's *Lady and the Tramp,* where the Italian restaurateurs are trying to create a romantic mood for the canine lovers in the back alley.

John and I weren't lovers, of course, but in the past two months we'd formed a unique bond of friendship that helped sustain us through the seemingly interminable nights when his friends and colleagues were being brought in to him in body bags. He trusted me and the rest of our team to handle his fellow Port Authority officers—and every other victim—as we would our own friends and family. But that night he revealed a deep hurt tinged with anger that I knew had been building for some time.

"You know, Emily," he went on, "we lost thirty-seven of our guys down there. No police agency in this country has ever lost that many. But nobody seems to really care anymore. When I drive by those billboards praising everybody *else,* it kinda hurts. And what about the civilian victims? Those poor people were also just doing their jobs."

I nodded and stared into my coffee. "People who work in the morgue also get used to being forgotten in the grand scheme of things," I said softly. "We deal with death all the time, but that doesn't mean we're immune to it. Most people think we are, though, so what can you do? You find some way to keep going, and you learn to accept that people from the outside will never know what we're dealing with in here."

"I know life ain't fair," John told me. "But this *really* isn't fair."

"No," I agreed. "But you know, there's one little bit of it that does make sense to me. I can see why the families need to be sheltered from the facts. If they actually knew what we had to deal with here, they'd have a clear idea of what happened to the people that died. I can see why they wouldn't want to know."

John laughed. "Silent servants," he said, quoting a phrase that one of the religious counselors liked to use. "Hidden heroes. That's us, all right."

I stretched my legs and thought about going back for more coffee, but I was just too comfortable where I was. "I wish I *was* a hero," I told him. "But I get so discouraged when I can't do more to help the families."

John and I sat there for a long time. We told each other that we were reluctant to go back out into the pouring rain. But I knew we were just basking in the glow of each other's company. He told me about his career in the Port Authority, his wife and children, and what had happened on the day he'd run for his life as the towers crashed down around him. I told him about my Kentucky cases, my family, and my little dog, Savannah, who I suspected was the only one who really missed me that night.

I still couldn't talk about my dad, and John respected that because he couldn't talk about how he felt, either, when one of his friends was brought to us in a body bag. We sat together for a long time that night. Then we went back to work.

•   •   •

It was a lonely time—but the New York City cops did everything they could to make me feel welcome. After that day on the pile, they treated me as one of their own, inviting me to hang out in their "private" tent and taking me up to Rockefeller Center to see the Christmas tree. Mark Grogan even brought me along to watch the Macy's Thanksgiving Day parade from his family's rented penthouse in the Mayflower Hotel.

Being pulled into the brotherhood of New York's Finest and Bravest wasn't just a social thing. Now that I felt the kinship, I shared their grief as well as their camaraderie. When the police or firefighters brought one of their own into the morgue, I was confronted with the living relatives of the dead—not just once, but several times a week—a kind of emotional demand that I hadn't dealt with before, as they entrusted me with their fellow members of service. I think it mattered, too, that I was obviously older than just about everyone else and usually the only woman handling the remains when they first came in, which made me a kind of emotional focus—almost a mother figure—for many of the men working at the site. If I was to do my job, I had to keep my scientist brain turned on, cataloguing, sorting, deducing, identifying. But if I was to honor the people with whom I worked, the people whose living bodies clustered around the dead remains, I had to allow my hands to channel the love and pain of every mother, wife, sister, and daughter of every one of the victims.

Still, feeling so much, night after night, week after week, took its toll. Sometimes I felt like a well that was about to run dry. My well-spun cocoon of defense was wearing thin, with even a hole here and there—but I kept working.

In the end, I think what made it all possible was knowing how much our efforts meant to the rest of the city—and to the country. Messages of thanks and well-wishing flowed into us from all over America, from schoolchildren and veterans' posts and police departments in other cities. I hope they could feel our appreciation flowing back to them.

I wanted a perfect ending. Now I've learned, the hard way, that some poems don't rhyme and some stories don't have a clear beginning, middle, and end. Life is about not knowing, having to change, taking the moment and making the best of it, without knowing what's going to happen next. Delicious Ambiguity.

— GILDA RADNER

Acknowledgments

I STAND ON THE SHOULDERS of those who came here first: the anthropologists, pathologists, and investigators who have devoted their lives and careers to the fascinating and sometimes heartbreaking world of forensic science. Without their care and guidance I would not have a place on the team. Without their continued help and support, this book could not have been written.

Mal Black, Octavia Garlington, and David Mascaro taught me how to marry art and science. The entire staff of the Hughston Sports Medicine Foundation and Clinic supported my career as a medical illustrator, while Dr. Jack C. Hughston taught me more than I ever wanted to know about the human knee. Dr. Bill Bass, founding father of forensic anthropology, brought me into his world with the determination to make sure that I learned his lessons well. Bill, I hope to make you proud.

I also hope this book conveys the respect and gratitude I have for my friends and colleagues in Kentucky's Justice Cabinet. In particular, I want to thank Dr. George Nichols and David Jones, who first laid the groundwork for Kentucky's Division of Medical Examiners, as well as Dr. Tracey Corey, who courageously tries to steer me and the rest of the staff to carry on the dream. All the support staff, pathologists, coroners, law enforcement officers, attorneys, judges, and juries working together to bring justice to this world have a special place in my heart. Of course, all the views expressed here and the perception of events are entirely my own.

This book is also the result of superhuman efforts on the part of my writing and publishing team. Special thanks must go to Rachel Kranz, whose genius helped turn my country girl's stories into a manuscript full of procedural drama, and to my agent, Jeff Kleinman, who, with extraordinary effort and talent, polished my work enough to take it to Crown Publishers. There I was lucky enough to have two editors, Emily Loose and Rachel Kahan, devote a huge amount of time and effort to the manuscript. Their skill and dedication are evident on every page. Heartfelt thanks as well to the rest of Crown's team: publisher Steve Ross, associate editor Caroline Sincerbeaux, production editor Jim Walsh, copy editor Steve Samuels, interior designer Lenny Henderson, and production manager Linnea Knollmueller.

Finally I wish to acknowledge the memory of my dear cousin, Jerry Hurley, whose bullet-ridden and decomposed body was found in the woods beside an abandoned Indiana gravel pit. May he rest in peace.

ABOUT THE AUTHOR

EMILY A. CRAIG, Ph.D., is the forensic anthropologist for the Commonwealth of Kentucky and one of the world's foremost forensic anthropologists. In addition to her work in Kentucky, she regularly consults with prosecutors, attorneys, police departments, and other law enforcement agencies from around the world, and she is a consultant to the United Nations Mission in Kosovo.

After earning her master's degree in medical illustration from the Medical College of Georgia in 1976, Dr. Craig worked at the Hughston Sports Medicine Foundation in Columbus, Georgia. Her groundbreaking studies earned her a worldwide reputation as an expert in the surgical anatomy of the musculoskeletal system. During this career in orthopedics, Dr. Craig illustrated and helped author hundreds of scientific articles and medical textbooks. She created numerous scientific exhibits for presentation all across the United States and Europe and pioneered techniques that combined her knowledge of art, anatomy, and computer graphics.

Dr. Craig then stepped away from this career to enter the world of forensic anthropology. Under the tutelage of Dr. Bill Bass, she earned her doctorate in the prestigious Forensic Physical Anthropology program at the University of Tennessee at Knoxville. Here she became one of the few forensic scientists in the world to undertake extensive research at the infamous "Body Farm," a secluded facility dedicated to the study and documentation of human decay processes.

Since beginning her second career as a full-time forensic anthropologist, Dr. Craig has developed an international reputation as an expert in the identification and analysis of human remains, and she has published numerous scientific articles and textbook chapters dealing with these subjects. Her prodigious work has earned her a coveted place among the ranks of fewer than sixty board-certified forensic anthropologists in the United States, and it continues to put her on the front lines of the world's most baffling mysteries.